Annales Nestlé

Cholestatic Disease in Childhood

Editor
Jacques Schmitz, Paris

S. Karger
Medical and Scientific Publishers
Basel · Freiburg · Paris ·
London · New York ·
Bangalore · Bangkok · Shanghai ·
Singapore · Tokyo · Sydney

KARGER

Nestlé Nutrition
INSTITUTE

S. Karger
Medical and Scientific Publishers
Basel • Freiburg • Paris • London
New York • Bangalore • Bangkok
Shanghai • Singapore • Tokyo • Sydney

P.O. Box, CH–4009 Basel (Switzerland)
Printed in Switzerland on acid-free paper by
Reinhardt Druck, Basel (Switzerland)
ISBN 978–3–8055–8965–9

KARGER

Fax +41 61 306 12 34
E-Mail karger@karger.ch
www.karger.com

Vol. 66, No. 3, 2008

Annales Nestlé

Contents

107 **Editorial**

109 **Diagnosis of Neonatal Cholestasis**
Girard, M.; Lacaille, F. (Paris)

121 **Familial Cholestatic Syndromes**
Thompson, R. (London)

127 **Treatments in Chronic Cholestasis in Children**
Alvarez, F. (Montreal, Qué.)

137 **Nutritional Management of Cholestatic Syndromes in Childhood**
Socha, P. (Warsaw)

KARGER

Fax +41 61 306 12 34
E-Mail karger@karger.ch
www.karger.com

Access to full text and tables of contents,
including tentative ones for forthcoming issues:
www.karger.com/ane_issues

Policy Statement

The Nestlé Nutrition Institute was created to provide health professionals with up to date information on nutrition and nutrition-related disorders in order to enable them to continuously improve patient care based on the latest medical and scientific breakthroughs.

One of the key pillars of the Nestlé Nutrition Institute is the *Annales Nestlé*, a pediatric journal that has been published on a regular basis since 1942. It contains review articles on clinical practice and research in all fields of pediatrics with focus on nutrition. Each publication deals with one specific topic, such as diabetes mellitus, HIV and nutrition or infant growth. The *Annales Nestlé* comprises 3 issues each year in 4 languages (English, French, Spanish and German), and with around 70,000 copies per issue is one of the most widely read pediatric journals in the world.

The *Annales Nestlé* is edited by an independent editorial board of six highly respected professors of pediatrics, thus guaranteeing the medical and scientific impartiality of the journal, and hence the high level of respect and appreciation in medical and scientific circles. The editorial board sets editorial policy, identifies topics to be addressed, selects authors and assesses the articles' contents.

The *Annales Nestlé* are published by S. Karger AG, one of the world's most highly respected scientific and medical publishers.

Prof. Ferdinand Haschke, MD, PhD
Chairman
Nestlé Nutrition Institute
Vevey (Switzerland)

KARGER
Fax +41 61 306 12 34
E-Mail karger@karger.ch
www.karger.com

Access to full text and tables of contents,
including tentative ones for forthcoming issues:
www.karger.com/ane_issues

Annales Nestlé

Ann Nestlé [Engl] 2008;66:107–108
DOI: 10.1159/000147407

Editorial

Cholestasis may be defined physiologically as a reduction in canalicular bile flow. Although it is clinically manifested as jaundice due to conjugated hyperbilirubinemia, its main consequences are due, on the one hand, to the cellular toxicity of accumulated bile acids, ultimately leading to biliary cirrhosis and, on the other hand, to decreased intraluminal bile acid concentration responsible for fat and fat-soluble vitamin malabsorption. Because the hepatobiliary excretory system is functionally immature at birth, the neonate has a particular tendency to develop cholestasis. Indeed, cholestatic diseases have been central in the development of pediatric hepatology. Around biliary atresia, the main cause of cholestasis in infants, multiple other causes have been recognized, related either to anatomic or genetic anomalies or to infectious or toxic agents, with very different prognoses.

Several reasons justify why this issue of *Annales Nestlé* is dedicated to cholestasis in childhood:

(1) impressive progresses have been made in the past 10 years in the characterization of several genetic defects affecting biliary secretion at the molecular level as well as in the clinical evaluation of their treatment and prognosis;

(2) on clinical grounds, the difficulty remains to recognize cholestasis and identify, as early as possible, a cause that could be amenable to medical therapy (e.g., galactosemia, inborn error of bile acid synthesis) or to early surgical intervention (biliary atresia) for an infant presenting with various degrees of jaundice, dark urines, pale or acholic stools and often hepatomegaly;

(3) early and adapted medical interventions may avoid the need for liver transplantation which, although life saving, remains a difficult procedure, with frequent side effects.

This background explains the selection of topics covered in this issue.

The first article, by Muriel Girard and Florence Lacaille from the Department of Pediatric Gastroenterology, Hepatology and Nutrition at Necker-Enfants Malades University Hospital, Paris, France, is logically devoted to the diagnosis of cholestasis, mainly in neonates, because it is at that age that it is crucial to ascertain or eliminate biliary atresia as early as possible. Their vast clinical experience allows them to write a comprehensive chapter ending with useful diagnostic algorithms and basic advice on how not to miss biliary atresia.

Then, Dr. Richard Thompson, Senior Lecturer in Paediatric Hepatology at King's College London School of Medicine, London, UK, well known for his studies on the genetics of progressive familial intrahepatic cholestasis, describes the various genetic defects affecting biliary secretion. He explains clearly why certain conditions are multisystem disorders whereas others are confined to the liver, according to the organ expression of the gene involved, and how the prognosis is linked to the genetic defect, particularly in the case of bile sort export pump deficiency whose prognosis is darkened by the risk of hepatocellular carcinoma. Of additional interest, this chapter highlights the relations between clinical phenotype and genotype and, more specifically, demonstrates that knowing the genetic cause of a disease makes it easier to identify phenotype variations.

KARGER

Fax +41 61 306 12 34
E-Mail karger@karger.ch
www.karger.com

0517–8606/08/0663–0107$24.50/0

Accessible online at:
www.karger.com/ane

Once the correct diagnosis is made, the adapted treatment should be initiated; this is the subject of the last 2 articles.

In his chapter, Dr. Fernando Alvarez, Professor of Pediatrics at Saint Justine University Hospital, University of Montreal, Montreal, Canada, senior pediatric hepatologist, deals with the specific treatments available for children with chronic cholestasis, emphasizing that very few of its causes have a specific treatment and that in most cases, therapeutic medical or surgical strategies are aimed at preventing or treating complications of bile (mostly bile acids) retention. The unique role of ursodeoxycholic acid in improving cholestasis is well explained; its rapid efficacy on liver tests is stressed as well as our ignorance of the benefit of its long-term administration. In addition to the drugs used to treat pruritus and malabsorption, the place of surgical procedures is well described and the necessity of an early Kasai intervention again underlined.

Because of the nutritional risks linked to chronic cholestasis and the importance of a good nutritional status when liver transplantation is envisaged, it is logical that the last chapter of the issue deals with the nutritional management of cholestatic syndromes in childhood. Dr. Piotr Socha, Professor of Pediatrics at the Children's Memorial Health Institute in Warsaw, Poland, an expert in nutrition in this field, has written a comprehensive review of the causes of malnutrition in these children, the diagnosis of specific deficiencies and of their treatment. The importance of bringing to these children enough protein and energy to achieve catch-up growth, either orally, by tube feeding or even by a central line, is well stressed as is the necessity of following the lipid-soluble vitamin status to correct possible deficiencies. The difficulties in polyunsaturated fatty acid and vitamin E supplementation are emphasized.

This issue does not deal with liver transplantation because, although an often necessary life-saving end-stage treatment of some of the causes of cholestasis in childhood, it represents another chapter in the story of these diseases, a chapter that is postponed as long as possible.

On the contrary, some of the congenital causes of cholestasis are a good example of conditions where the knowledge of their genetic defect may lead to new therapeutic strategies such as gene therapy or hepatocyte transplantation.

The Editorial Committee

Annales Nestlé

Ann Nestlé [Engl] 2008;66:109–120
DOI: 10.1159/000147408

Diagnosis of Neonatal Cholestasis

Muriel Girard Florence Lacaille

Pediatric Gastroenterology-Hepatology-Nutrition Unit, Necker-Enfants Malades Hospital, Paris, France

Key Words
Neonatal cholestasis · Acholic stools · Biliary atresia · Metabolic disease

Abstract
Cholestasis is frequent in neonates (1/2,500 live births) and in young children. It includes many etiologies with sometimes poor prognosis. In case of neonatal cholestasis, the most important point is to look at the stool color and to rule out biliary atresia which needs to be surgically treated before the 45th day of life. Biliary atresia represents almost 50% of cases of neonatal cholestasis, the other causes being numerous. Some cases can be treated with success, such as tyrosinemia type I or inborn errors of bile acid synthesis. However, in the majority of cases, there is no specific treatment, and the evolution of the disease is toward cirrhosis or liver insufficiency leading to liver transplantation. Nowadays, liver transplantation has good results, but it is a difficult procedure with frequent side effects. In the future, analysis and a better understanding of the mechanisms of the different cholestatic diseases could allow the development of other treatments such as liver cell transplantation or gene therapy, bringing new perspectives for children.

Introduction

Cholestasis in children often appears in the first weeks of life, because the neonate is particularly predisposed by the biliary secretion immaturity. Neonatal cholestasis is frequent and its incidence is 1/2,500 live births. The identification of the cause of cholestasis is very important, because the most frequent one is biliary atresia which should be corrected surgically before 45 days of life [1]. Many other diseases can lead to cholestasis in the neonatal period. Moreover, 15 diseases account for 95% of cases, and the prognosis depends on the etiology. Cholestasis is the most frequent cause of liver transplantation in children, and liver transplantation dramatically changes the prognosis. Currently, an increasing number of genes involved in diseases causing neonatal cholestasis are known, and identification of a pathological mutation in a family can allow prenatal diagnosis for the more severe diseases. Also, in the future, identification of other genes involved in these diseases will lead to a better understanding of the mechanisms of cholestasis, and, probably, to new therapies other than liver transplantation.

Physiopathology of Cholestasis

Cholestasis is defined by manifestations linked to diminished or absent bile flux or by abnormal bile formation. It can be due to metabolic hepatocyte alterations

KARGER

Fax +41 61 306 12 34
E-Mail karger@karger.ch
www.karger.com

0517–8606/08/0663–0109$24.50/0

Accessible online at:
www.karger.com/ane

Muriel Girard
Pediatric Gastroenterology-Hepatology-Nutrition Unit
Necker-Enfants Malades Hospital, 149 rue de Sèvres
FR–75015 Paris (France)
E-Mail muriel.girard@nck.aphp.fr

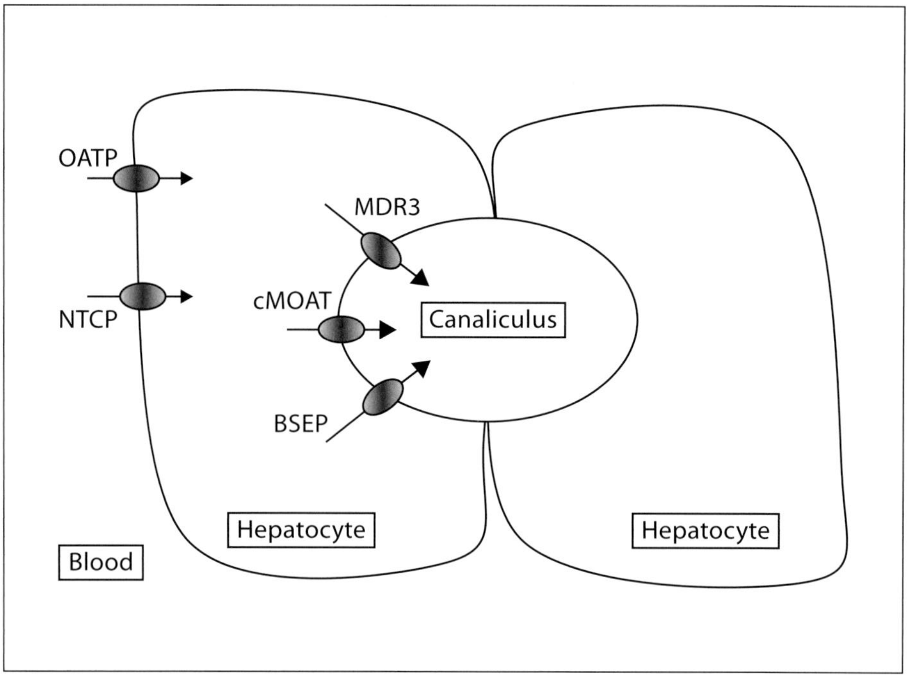

Fig. 1. Main steps of bile production in the hepatocyte. Bile production is an active process, involving the transport of bile acids and other osmotic compounds across a concentration gradient into the bile canaliculus. At the apical pole of hepatocyte: OATP = Organic anion transporting protein; NTCP = Na taurocholate cotransporting polypeptide. At the canaliculus pole of hepatocyte: cMOAT = Canalicular multispecific organic anion transporter; BSEP = bile salt export pump; MDR3 = multidrug resistance protein 3.

(secondary to hepatocyte injury or to external factors such as infection or parenteral nutrition) or to intra- or extrahepatic biliary alterations.

Bile production is an active process, involving the transport of bile acids and other osmotic compounds across a concentration gradient into the bile canaliculus. This osmotic concentration induces the passive movement of water into the canaliculus. Active transporters are localized at the basolateral membrane of the hepatocyte for sinusoidal blood uptake (fig. 1): Na taurocholate cotransporting polypeptide (NTCP), organic anion transporting protein (OATP) and, at the canalicular membrane for biliary excretion, bile salt export pump (BSEP), canalicular multispecific organic anion transporter (cMOAT) and multidrug resistance protein 3 (MDR3). The expression of these transporters is modified by liver disease, injury or sepsis in order to protect the hepatocyte from the cytotoxic effects of elevated bile acid concentration. This regulation could probably explain why jaundice may be an early sign of sepsis. Bile flow is low in the fetus and newborn because of the immaturity of bile acid synthesis and transport processes. In animal models, NTCP and BSEP are present already before birth, but at a very low level in comparison with adults. The development process for human hepatocyte transporters has not yet been quantified, but plasma bile acids do not fall into the normal adult range until 6 months of age. These observations strongly suggest the predisposition of the neonate to cholestasis [2, 3].

Diagnosis of Cholestasis

Cholestasis should be suspected if jaundice has not disappeared during the second week of life. Cholestatic jaundice is associated with pale stools and dark urines; there is no pruritus in the neonatal period. The liver may be enlarged, firm or hard. Sometimes, a splenomegaly is present. Acholic stools, hard liver and abdominal or thoracic situs inversus are very suggestive of biliary atresia. Biological features of cholestasis are hyperbilirubinemia, mainly conjugated, and often elevated γ-glutamyl transferase, as well as alkaline phosphatase activities and serum bile salts. It is important to differentiate jaundice of liver insufficiency and a cholestatic jaundice (in this situation, prothrombin time is normalized after vitamin K_1 injection). In cholestasis, there is liposoluble vitamin malabsorption and vitamin K_1 deficiency, predisposing to bleeding; an injection of vitamin K_1 should always be performed. Abdominal ultrasonography should be performed in all cholestatic infants, by an experienced radiologist. Intrahepatic bile ducts are rarely dilated, suggesting gallstone or a choledocal cyst. A small and dysmorphic gallbladder is very suggestive of biliary atresia, but is not specific, because the gallbladder is empty when the cholestasis is severe. On the contrary, a normal gallbladder does not exclude biliary atresia, because of cystic forms of biliary atresia. The aim is not to miss biliary atresia. The diagnostic procedure should be performed as quickly as possible. If the stools are permanently acholic, a liver biopsy or a cholangiography must be performed to rule out or confirm biliary atresia.

Etiologies

Extrahepatic Diseases

Exclusively extrahepatic causes of neonatal cholestasis are rare (5%) and can easily be diagnosed by ultrasonography. The stools may be permanently or transiently acholic.

Lithiasis of the common bile duct may cause severe cholestasis, and the presentation may be intermittent acholic stools. Predisposing factors are hyperhemolysis or parenteral nutrition. Spontaneous elimination of the calculus is frequent. On the contrary, a percutaneous cholecystography can allow to wash out the stone. In principle, there is no recurrence.

Spontaneous perforation of the bile duct is very rare and occurs often at the junction of the common bile duct and cystic duct. Clinical presentation is biliary peritonitis, bile collection or biliary stenosis. The treatment is surgical.

A choledochal cyst is rarely discovered in the neonatal period, but is the second most frequent surgical cause of neonatal cholestasis. In the neonatal period, the clinical presentation is usually similar to biliary atresia, but can also be a sudden onset of cholestasis or cholangitis with abdominal pain and pancreatitis. The diagnosis is made by ultrasonography or tomodensitometry. The treatment is surgical with total ablation of the residual cyst to avoid later malignant transformation. The long-term prognosis is very good, with a normal liver function.

Extra- and Intrahepatic Causes

Biliary Atresia

Biliary atresia is the most frequent cause of neonatal cholestasis and accounts for almost 50% of cases. It is the first indication of liver transplantation in children. The incidence is 1/10,000 live births. It results from a bile duct obliteration beginning in utero or in the very early postnatal period. The bile duct alteration (inflammatory destruction) involves the whole biliary tree in 80% of cases. The cause of biliary atresia is still unknown, but a genetic origin can be suspected in some cases because of the association of some heterotaxic elements such as abdominal or thoracic situs inversus, and polyspleny in about 20% of cases, and a high incidence (×6) in some populations [4]. The aim of the surgery is to re-establish a bile flow through an intestinal loop (Kasai procedure). It will be successful if the intrahepatic bile ducts at the hilum are not yet occluded. Because the inflammatory destruction seems to be progressive, the Kasai procedure should be performed as early as possible. Before 45 days of life, the child has an 80% chance of remaining without jaundice at the age of 3 years. If the Kasai procedure is performed after 45 days of life, the success of the surgery decreases dramatically. If the Kasai procedure fails, the evolution of the disease is toward biliary cirrhosis, and a liver transplantation has to be performed between 1 and 2 years of life. Even when the Kasai procedure is efficient, in a large majority of cases, cirrhosis is already present, with a risk of portal hypertension and intestinal bleeding. The child can also develop cholangitis, icterus and chronic liver insufficiency, as well as acute liver failure; a liver transplantation is often necessary later on. Only 10% of children are alive without liver transplant at the age of 20 years [5]. Because of the severity and the importance of early diagnosis, biliary atresia should systematically be suspected in neonatal cholestasis. The diagnosis is strongly suspected if the child permanently has acholic stools (particularly from birth) with a hard hepatomegaly, if there are heterotaxic elements, if there is a biliary cyst at the hilum, and if the gallbladder is small and dysmorphic after fasting. Ultrasonography can help the diagnosis, but the diagnosis is actually made by cholangiography realized either at a laparoscopy or directly at laparotomy, both followed with the Kasai procedure if necessary.

Neonatal Sclerosing Cholangitis

Neonatal sclerosing cholangitis is a very rare disease, different from primary sclerosing cholangitis as seen in older children and associated with inflammatory bowel disease. The clinical presentation is a severe neonatal cholestasis, with acholic stools, that can mimic biliary atresia. The diagnosis is made by cholangiography, which shows patent intrahepatic ducts but irregular narrowing of extrahepatic or intrahepatic bile ducts. Usually, no intestinal disease is found in these patients. Frequently, there is a resolution of the icterus, but early cirrhosis and portal hypertension; a liver transplantation is necessary for few children [6]. Some observations suggest a genetic origin because of familial cases [7]. A few cases associated with ichthyosis are linked to a mutation in the *Claudin-1* gene, encoding for a tight-junction molecule [8]. Other cases of this neonatal ichthyosis-sclerosing cholangitis (NISCH) syndrome have been described and show a variable clinical expression in the skin and liver phenotype [9]. However, the majority of children with neonatal sclerosing cholangitis have no ichthyosis, suggesting that the disease is heterogeneous.

Sclerosing Cholangitis with Postnatal Onset

Cholangitis can be associated with other diseases such as histiocytosis X, immunodeficiency syndrome, chronic inflammatory bowel disease or autoimmune hepatitis and congenital psoriasis. However, in some cases, there is no associated disease [6].

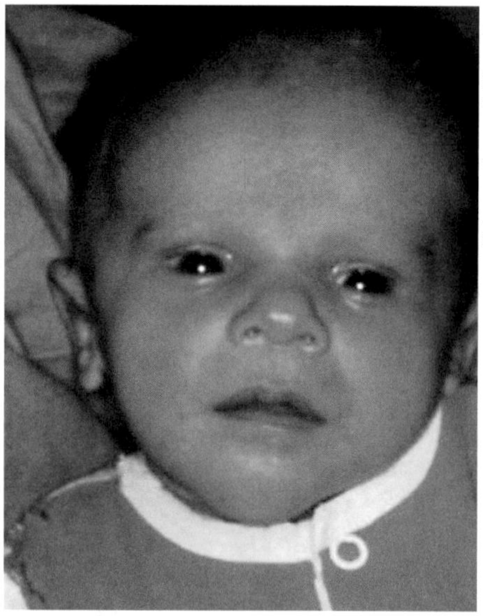

Color version available online

Fig. 2. Picture of an infant with Alagille syndrome. Note the typical features: prominent forehead, deep-set eyes, hypertelorism, small pointed chin.

Intrahepatic Causes

Intrahepatic cholestasis represents almost 50% of the causes of neonatal cholestasis and comprises a heterogeneous group of diseases.

Infectious Diseases

The classical causes are fetopathies (congenital rubella, toxoplasmosis, cytomegalovirus and syphilis infections), often associated with a low birth weight, neurological or hematological symptoms. Bacterial infections (the most frequent is urinary tract infection with *Escherichia coli*) can induce inhibition of canalicular bile acid transport and cause cholestasis.

Toxic Causes

The most frequent toxic agent for the liver in the neonatal period is parenteral nutrition. The mechanisms are probably complex, associating recurrent infections, inflammatory response, inappropriate content of the parenteral nutrition, absence of enterohepatic circulation and immaturity of bile transport [10]. In some cases, children with very severe cholestasis induced by parenteral nutrition may develop liver failure. Drug injury can be an additional factor to liver alterations. A polymorphism associated with a decreased hepatic *BSEP* expression was significantly more frequent in drug-induced cholestasis in adult patients [11], suggesting that genetic factors could also play a role in neonates in inducing parenteral nutrition liver disease.

Ischemia

Ischemia in newborns is frequently accompanied by cholestasis, without symptoms other than uncomplicated cholestasis. Cholestasis is associated with several contributing factors related to the severity of the neonatal distress. Neonates born before the age of 35 weeks have an increased risk (×3) of neonatal cholestasis [12, 13].

Genetic Diseases

Alagille Syndrome

Alagille syndrome is an autosomal dominant disorder also called 'syndromic bile duct hypoplasia'. It affects all ethnic groups. It is characterized by neonatal jaundice, intrahepatic cholestasis and developmental disorders affecting the liver, heart, vertebra, eyes and face. Alagille syndrome represents 10–15% of neonatal cholestasis, and its frequency is 1/100,000 live births. The clinical diagnosis is made on the association of facial dysmorphy (prominent forehead, deep-set eyes, hypertelorism, small pointed chin; fig. 2), posterior embryotoxon, butterfly-shaped vertebra, peripheral stenosis of the pulmonary artery (or another cardiopathy), and cholestasis due to paucity of the interlobular bile ducts. The inheritance is dominant, with a variable penetrance and a great heterogeneity in clinical manifestations, suggesting that several factors are important in the pathogenesis. The prognosis is worse in children who present with neonatal cholestatic jaundice, with rare resolution of jaundice. A majority of them will require liver transplantation in childhood [14]. However, severe liver complications are also possible in late-onset liver disease, requiring follow-up throughout life. A molecular diagnosis is possible: 70% of patients have a mutation in the *jagged-1* gene encoding for a Notch receptor involved in cellular differentiation and development. The mechanism is probably haploinsufficiency. There is no genotype-phenotype correlation. No clustering was observed, and the majority of mutations are familial specific mutations. Sporadic cases are the most frequent (70%) relative to the high rate of de novo mutations [15]. There is a high rate of new mutations that makes the molecular diagnosis difficult.

α_1-Antitrypsine Deficiency

α_1-Antitrypsine deficiency is a common recessive disorder, affecting 1/2,000 live births. The diagnosis is suggested by protein electrophoresis with an absent pic of α-globulins and confirmed by the specific dosage of serum α_1-antitrypsine and phenotype protein analysis. The α_1-antitrypsine protein is synthesized in the liver and exported to the lung. In the lung, the protein functions as an antiprotease, preventing alveolar damage caused by leukocyte elastase. The abnormal protein has a 'Z' phenotype and cannot be exported out of the liver and polymerizes in the endoplasmic reticulum. Intrahepatic accumulation of the mutant Z protein in the liver induces activation of autophagy, mitochondrial injury and caspase activation, and thus, hepatocellular injury. Only patients with the ZZ genotype develop cholestasis in childhood or lung and liver disease in adulthood. Liver disease can occur at any age. The majority of children are free of significant liver dysfunction, and only a small proportion of homozygous ZZ children (10–15%) develop cholestasis in the neonatal period. The variable clinical presentation suggests an important contribution of genetic and environmental modifiers. The heterozygous carrier state for the mutant Z gene, present in 1.5–3% of the population, is not a cause of liver injury but may be a modifier gene for other liver diseases [16–18]. The clinical feature of neonatal presentation can be very similar to biliary atresia. There is no specific management and the outcome is variable: 50% of children will no longer have liver abnormality in adulthood, 10% will remain cholestatic and require liver transplantation, and some of the children (40–50%) have a compensated liver disease with mild alterations and may require liver transplantation in adulthood.

Cystic Fibrosis

Cystic fibrosis is one of the most frequent hereditary diseases in Caucasians (1/2,000 live births in Europe). The clinical presentation may be variable. Neonatal cholestasis is a typical but rare primary clinical manifestation in cystic fibrosis and is most often associated with meconium ileus. The mechanism is probably obstruction of bile ductules by abnormal mucoid secretions. Patients may have complete cholestasis, mimicking biliary atresia. In cystic fibrosis patients with neonatal cholestasis, one third have another condition, increasing the risk of cholestasis, such as α_1-antitrypsin deficiency, hypopituitarism, perinatal asphyxia and total parenteral nutrition [19].

Progressive Familial Intrahepatic Cholestasis

Progressive familial intrahepatic cholestasis (PFIC) is a heterogeneous group of diseases that accounts for 10% of neonatal cholestasis. The clinical presentation is neonatal or childhood cholestasis with pruritus. The evolution is cirrhosis or liver insufficiency in childhood, often requiring liver transplantation. The inheritance is autosomal recessive. Three groups of diseases have recently been identified, with particular phenotypic features (see the following chapter).

PFIC-1 and PFIC-2 are characterized by early cholestasis with a frequent liver insufficiency and severe pruritus; the gamma GT activity is always normal. PFIC-1 is due to a mutation in the *FIC1* gene, encoding for an ATPase, present at the canalicular pole of the hepatocyte and playing a still unknown role in bile formation. Some patients may have impairment of other organs except for the liver, such as diarrhea, renal failure, pancreatitis and deafness. PFIC-2 is due to a mutation in the *BSEP* gene which is implicated in the export of bile salts in the canaliculi. The evolution is often more severe than in the PFIC-1 deficiency.

PFIC-3, due to a mutation in the *MDR3* gene, is a transmembrane hepatocyte phospholipid transporter. Compared with the first 2 diseases, PFIC-3 deficiency is characterized by less pruritus, frequent portal hypertension, late liver insufficiency and high gamma GT activity.

Half of the patients with PFIC have a good response to ursodeoxycholic acid. Some children may benefit from a treatment with partial external biliary diversion (exept those with MDR3 deficiency). Partial responders or nonresponders will require liver transplantation [20–22]. If a molecular diagnosis is available for the family, a prenatal diagnosis is possible in some laboratories [23].

Inborn Errors of Bile Acid Synthesis

Inborn errors of bile acid synthesis are specific defects in the enzymes involved in the reactions leading from cholesterol to cholic and chenodeoxycholic acids [24]. At birth or in early childhood, affected individuals present with cholestatic jaundice, fat-soluble vitamin deficiency and acholic or fatty stools (steatorrhea). Serum transaminases are usually elevated, gamma GT activity is normal, and a conjugated hyperbilirubinemia is often present. Liver biopsies may reveal nonspecific changes, but giant cell transformation of hepatocytes, inflammation, fibrosis gamma GT activity is normal and canalicular and hepatocyte cholestasis are usual. Recognition of defects in bile acid synthesis relies upon mass spectrometric analysis of the urine and serum to establish an absence or marked reduction in certain primary bile acids, cholic and chenodeoxycholic acids, concomitant with the presence of excessive amounts of atypical bile acids and sterols, synthesized as a consequence of the enzyme deficiency.

Mutations of several genes have so far been identified (fig. 3) [25, 26]:

3β-hydroxy-C27-steroid dehydrogenase oxydoreductase deficiency (HSD3B7); Δ4-3-oxosteroid 5β-reductase deficiency (AKR1D1); oxysterol 7α-hydroxylase deficiency (CYP7B1); 2-methylacyl-CoA racemase deficiency; sterol 27-hydroxylase deficiency (CYP27A1); bile acid-CoA:amino acid N-acyltransferase deficiency (BAAT); cholesterol 7α-hydroxylase deficiency (CYP7A1).

Early diagnosis is important because patients can be successfully treated with oral administration of cholic acid. Normalization in serum liver enzymes and bilirubin and resolution of the histologic lesion are consistent responses to bile acid therapy, and the need for liver transplantation in most cases can be circumvented. Bile acid biosynthetic defects, in particular 3β-hydroxy-C27-steroid dehydrogenase oxydoreductase deficiency, may also cause late-onset chronic cholestasis; in these individuals, the clinical history generally reveals a pattern of mildly elevated transaminases in infancy, that often resolved, only to reappear later on with an early-onset of vitamin-D-deficient rickets.

Niemann-Pick Disease Type C

Niemann-Pick disease type C is a rare autosomal recessive lipid storage disorder characterized by progressive neurodegeneration. The clinical presentation is heterogeneous, and the age at onset varies between the perinatal period and adulthood. In the neonate, hepatomegaly and splenomegaly are frequent, associated with prolonged cholestatic jaundice. Usually, the icterus disappears spontaneously, but sometimes, a rapidly fatal liver failure develops. The age at onset of neurological symptoms and their evolution determine the severity of the disease. Niemann-Pick disease is found in 8% of infants evaluated for cholestasis; it should be considered in all infants with cholestasis, particularly those with splenomegaly or associated neurological symptoms. The diagnosis is suspected when lipid-laden foam cells are found in the bone marrow and liver. The mutated gene is involved in intracellular cholesterol transport and causes accumulation of nonesterified cholesterol in lysosomes. The diagnosis is established by demonstrating these anomalies in cultured fibroblasts. Molecular diagnosis is possible. Two genes are involved: *NPC1* and *NPC2*, allowing a prenatal diagnosis [27]. There is no specific treatment.

Mitochondrial Disorders

Mitochondrial disorders may manifest as neonatal acute liver failure, steatohepatitis, cholestasis or cirrhosis with chronic liver failure of insidious onset. Usually, there are significant neuromuscular symptoms, multisystem involvement and lactic acidemia. The liver disease is usually progressive and eventually fatal. Several molecular defects (mutations in nuclear genes such as *SCO1, BCS1L, POLG, DGUOK* and *MPV17* and deletion or rearrangement of mitochondrial DNA) have been identified in recent years with the possibility of genetic and prenatal diagnosis. Current medical therapy of mitochondrial hepatopathies is largely ineffective, and the prognosis is usually poor. The role of liver transplantation in patients with liver failure remains poorly defined because of the systemic nature of the disease with the possibility of the involvement of other organs than the liver [28, 29].

Galactosemia

Galactosemia is characterized by a deficiency in galactose metabolism resulting in the accumulation of galactose-1-phosphate. It is autosomal recessive and affects 1/35,000 births in Europe. The clinical symptoms appear during the first days of life and include vomiting, jaun-

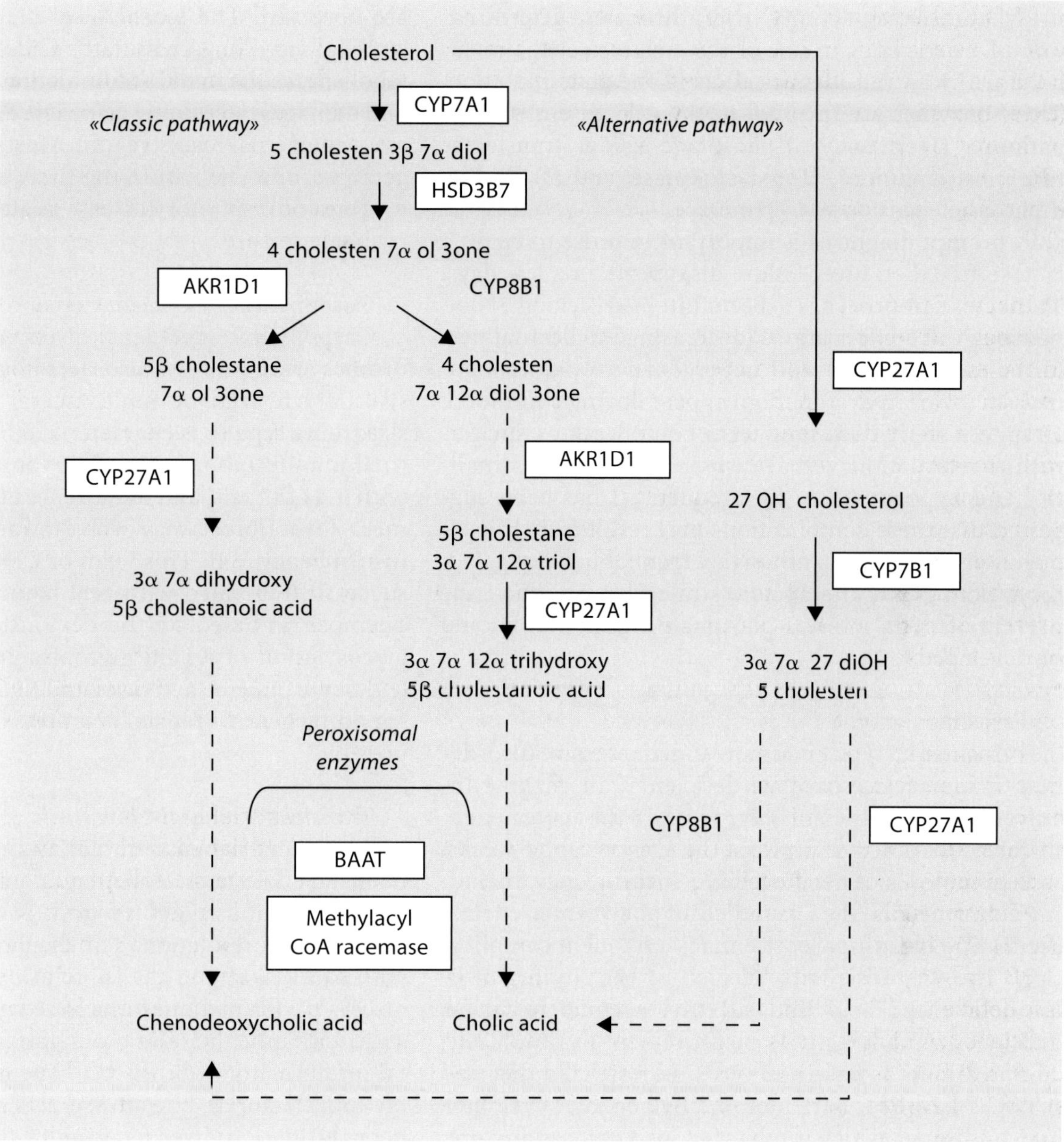

Fig. 3. Bile acid biosynthetic pathways. The classic pathway of bile acid biosynthesis is only present in hepatocytes. The alternative pathway exists in all tissues. Only major regulatory steps and enzymes are shown. The classic pathway synthesizes 2 primary bile acids, cholic acid and chenodeoxycholic acid. Framed enzymes are those known to be involved in inborn errors of bile acid synthesis. CYP7A1 = Cholesterol 7α-hydroxylase; HSD3B7 = 3β-hydroxyl Δ5-C27-steroid oxydoreductase; CYP8B1 = sterol 12α-hydroxylase; AKR1D1 = Δ4-3-oxosteroid 5β-reductase; CYP27A1 = sterol 27-hydroxylase; CYP7B1 = oxysterol 7α-hydroxylase; BAAT = bile acid CoA:amino acid-N-acyltransferase.

dice, lethargy, hepatomegaly, liver failure in a baby breastfed or receiving a lactose-containing formula. If left untreated, the condition evolves rapidly towards hepatic and renal failure with sepsis due to Gram-negative bacteria. Cataract develops after several days or weeks and becomes rapidly irreversible. The diagnosis relies on the detection of galactose-1-phosphate accumulation in erythrocytes (spot test), measurement of galactose-1-phosphate uridyl transferase activity in erythrocytes, determination of a deficiency in one of the enzymes of the metabolic pathway and identification of the gene mutation. Three enzymes are involved in the galactose metabolic pathway: (1) galactose-1-phosphate uridyl transferase (the most common), (2) galactokinase, and (3) uridine diphosphate galactose-4-epimerase.

A prompt diagnosis is important in order to begin a lactose-free diet. Liver failure disappears in a few days. The lactose-free diet has to be maintained lifelong. If not, neurological complications (decreasing intellectual performances with age) and hypergonadotropic hypogonadism (ovarian dysfunction) appear during childhood. Despite a strict diet, long-term complications such as mental retardation, verbal dyspraxia, motor abnormalities and hypogonadism are frequent. It has been suggested that these complications may result from the endogenous galactose synthesis or from abnormal galactosylation. Novel therapeutic strategies, aiming at the prevention of galactose-1-phosphate production, should be developed [30].

Tyrosinemia Type I

Tyrosinemia type I is an autosomal recessive disorder due to fumarylacetoacetate deficiency, an enzyme involved in the catabolism of tyrosine. In the acute neonatal form, onset occurs between the ages of 2 and 6 weeks, with symptoms of hepatocellular insufficiency, including vomiting, diarrhea, jaundice, hypoglycemia, edema, ascites and bleeding. Septicemia is a frequent complication. The diagnosis is confirmed by the finding of δ-aminolevulinic acid and succinyl acetone in urine, and by enzymatic activity measurement in fibroblasts. The treatment is based on tyrosine-restricted diet and NTBC [(2-nitro-4-trifluoromethylbenzoyl)-cyclohexane-1,3-dione], which inhibits tyrosine oxidase and prevents the accumulation of toxic succinyl acetone [31]. Despite this treatment, some patients develop hepatoma with elevated α-fetoprotein and require liver transplantation [32]. Prenatal diagnosis relies on metabolite assay, enzymatic study or screening for the mutation when it is known.

Peroxisomal Disorders

Many peroxisomal disorders have an impact on bile acid synthesis [33]. The Zellweger syndrome which is defined by a reduced number of peroxisomes is characterized by dysmorphic craniofacial features, profound hypotonia, seizures, as well as liver and renal dysfunctions. Hepatomegaly and cholestasis with progressive fibrosis are observed. The biochemical diagnosis relies on the study of very-long-chain fatty acids. This impaired metabolism results in the accumulation of toxic metabolites and damages developing cells. The disease is transmitted as an autosomal recessive trait. Most infants with Zellweger syndrome die within the first year of life secondary to apnea or respiratory disease related to infection or intractable seizure.

Carbohydrate-Deficient Glycoprotein Syndromes

Carbohydrate-deficient glycoprotein (CDG) syndromes are a group of disorders in glycoprotein synthesis characterized by multivisceral involvement. CDG syndrome type Ib is characterized by hepatic and intestinal manifestations (diarrhea, vomiting, hepatomegaly with liver fibrosis) and the absence of neurologic involvement. Liver fibrosis may evolve toward cirrhosis and liver insufficiency [34]. This form of CDG syndrome can be successfully treated with oral mannose. The biological diagnosis is based on the demonstration of abnormal glycosylation of serum glycoproteins, measurement of leukocyte enzyme activities and mutations in the corresponding genes. Prenatal diagnosis of CDG syndrome is possible.

Transient Neonatal Cholestasis

Transcient neonatal cholestasis represents 5–10% of neonatal cholestasis. It is often called 'neonatal hepatitis', but no infectious agent is found. The evolution is always good toward resolution. The diagnosis should be made with caution, after a careful follow-up. When a liver biopsy is performed, multinucleated giant cell hepatitis is seen, with mild ductular proliferation and moderate portal inflammatory fibrosis [35]. The mechanism is probably multifactorial: bile acid secretion immaturity in the neonatal period, liver fetal injury (ischemia, infection), long-time fasting (parenteral nutrition) and possibly genetic factors predisposing to cholestasis [36]. The other causes of neonatal cholestasis have to be ruled out before this diagnosis is retained.

Practical Approach in the Diagnosis of Neonatal Cholestasis

In cases of suspected cholestasis, the first and most important point to assess is the color of the stools. If the stools are acholic, biliary atresia must be diagnosed or ruled out. If an obstructive pathology of the extrahepatic biliary tree is ruled out, the diagnosis of biliary atresia is

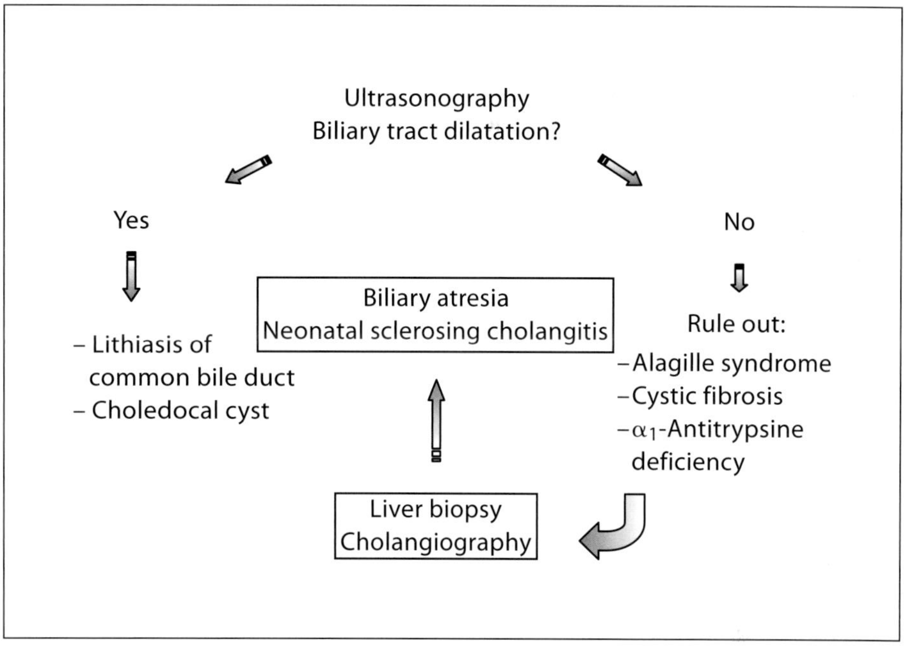

Fig. 4. Algorithm in the case of very pale or acholic stools. The first point is to know if the biliary tract is dilated or not. If there is no extrahepatic obstruction, Alagille syndrome, cystic fibrosis and α_1-antitrypsine deficiency must be ruled out. If no evident etiology is found, a liver biopsy or a cholangiography must be performed.

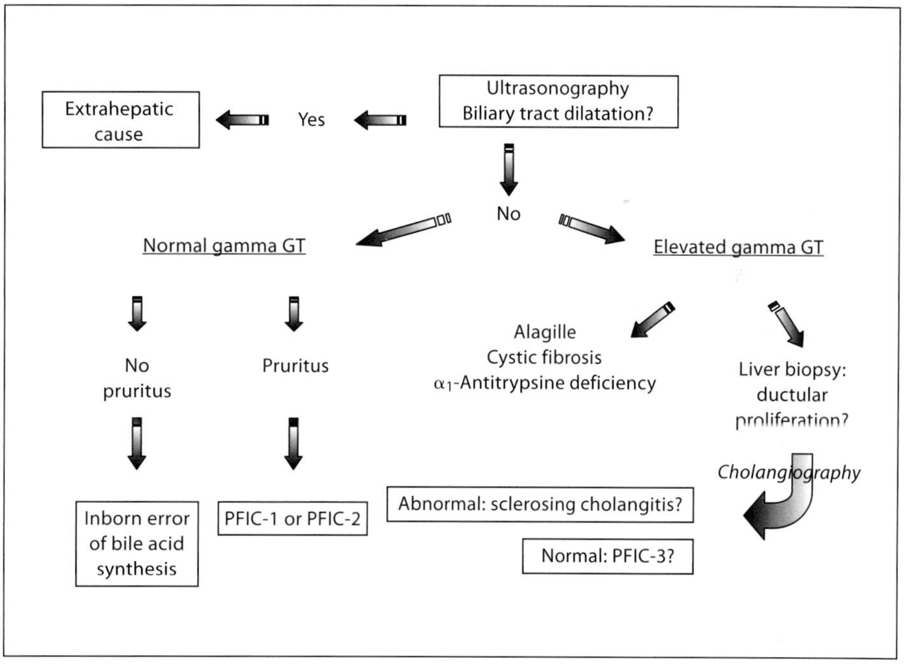

Fig. 5. Algorithm in the case of pale but not acholic stools. An extrahepatic obstacle must be ruled out. In cases of a low gamma GT level, a PFIC-1 or PFIC-2 and inborn errors of bile synthesis are possible. In cases of a high gamma GT level, Alagille syndrome, cystic fibrosis and α_1-antitrypsine deficiency must be ruled out. If no etiology is evident, a liver biopsy and cholangiography must be performed.

likely. A cholangiography and a liver biopsy must be performed. If the biliary tract is not patent, a Kasai procedure is to be performed. If the biliary tract is patent, another diagnosis and a possible neonatal sclerosing cholangitis have to be considered (fig. 4).

Biliary Atresia

In order not to miss biliary atresia, consider the following: (1) neonatal cholestasis is a biliary atresia until definitively demonstrated that it is not; (2) diagnosis of biliary atresia is an emergency; (3) do not first think of

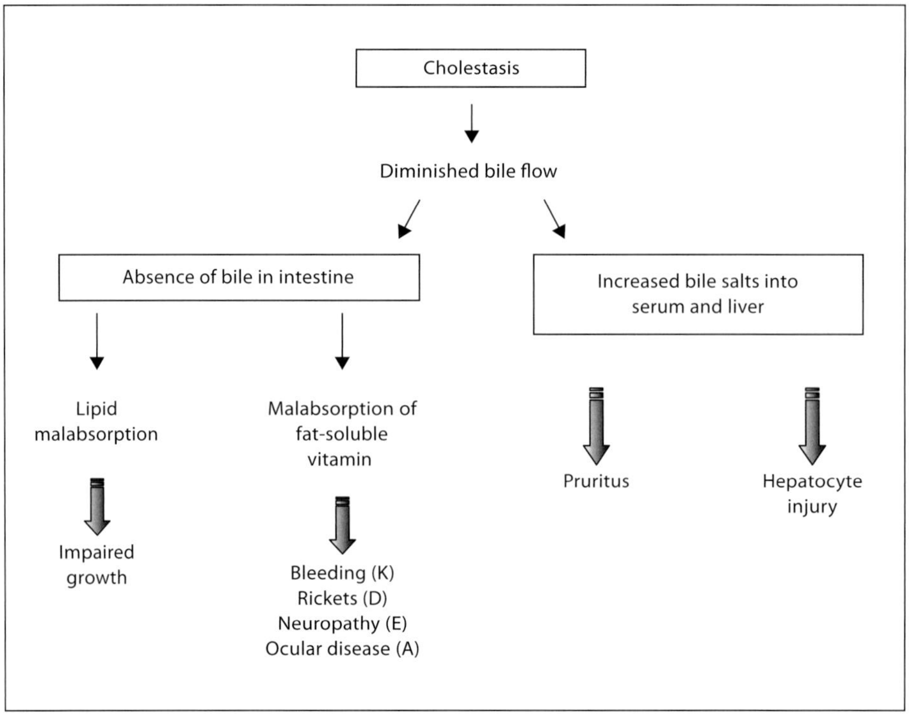

Fig. 6. Consequences of cholestasis. In cases of cholestasis, a diminished bile flow is responsible of an increase in serum bile salts leading to pruritus and liver injury. The absence of bile in the intestine leads to lipid malabsorption and impaired growth, and a fat-soluble vitamin malabsorption leads to bleeding (vitamin K deficiency), rickets (vitamin D deficiency), neuropathy (vitamin E deficiency) and ocular disease (vitamin A deficiency).

breast milk jaundice; (4) ask parents about the stool color; (5) do not think that a normal growth rules out a severe liver disease; (6) do not stop the explorations after finding cytomegalovirus in urines; (7) do not think that bilirubinemia is always very high in biliary atresia; (8) do a liver biopsy if the diagnosis is unclear; (9) organize an operative cholangiography when biliary atresia is not ruled out and the time is running.

If the stools are pale but not acholic, the biochemical tests (related to the various causes of neonatal cholestasis) or a liver biopsy will help the diagnosis. Different parameters are important, such as dilatation of the biliary tract and the level of gamma GT activity (fig. 5).

Management of a Cholestatic Child

In addition to a possible specific treatment, treatment of the consequences of cholestasis is important to avoid complications. The major consequence is the impairment of lipid absorption due to the absence of bile in the intestine. Malabsorption of fat-soluble vitamins may result in bleeding (vitamin K deficiency), rickets (vitamin D deficiency), neuropathy (vitamin E deficiency) and ocular disease (vitamin A deficiency). Fat-soluble vitamins should be given orally at large doses, as long as the cholestasis is not too severe and the level of vitamins A, E and D are checked regularly. If cholestasis is severe, or in case of poor response to the oral route, parenteral injections are mandatory.

Impaired lipid absorption and cholestasis may severely impair growth. Formulas enriched with medium-chain triglycerides may improve fat malabsorption and nutrition. In cholestatic infants, 180–200 calories/kg/day may be necessary, and enteral feeding could be used to maintain growth.

The use of ursodeoxycholic acid (a hydrophilic bile acid) is beneficial in cholestasis. The precise mechanisms of its action are not completely understood; there is probably an enrichment in the bile acid pool with more hydrophilic bile acids, and stimulation of bile flow. It improves biochemical parameters and controls fibrosis progression in PFIC. Its efficiency is not demonstrated in other cholestatic syndromes, but ursodeoxycholic acid seems to improve biochemical parameters and speeds the clearance of jaundice in transient neonatal cholestasis. The only side effect is diarrhea that responds to dose reduction. Its use is recommended at a dose of 20 mg/kg/day.

Pruritus is a debilitating symptom in severe cholestasis and is obvious only from the second semester of life. The most effective treatment is rifampicin, used at 5–20 mg/kg/day. The mechanism of action is unclear but probably involves the inhibition of hepatocyte bile uptake and the induction of microsomal enzymes. Phenobarbital and cholestyramine are less effective and have more side effects.

Vaccinations should be performed, especially if a liver transplantation is probable in the future (fig. 6).

Conclusion

The early diagnosis of neonatal cholestasis is important considering the severity of biliary atresia. Liver transplantation dramatically changed the prognosis of biliary atresia and a lot of other cholestatic diseases in children. Therapeutic progress in pediatric hepatology is essentially linked to liver transplantation that gives good chance of surviving and a good quality of life. The long-term results for transplantation are good, with a survival rate around 90%, 5 years after transplantation. But it is a very difficult procedure with a lot of surgical and medical complications such as renal insufficiency and posttransplant lymphoproliferative disease. Specific medical treatments have been developed in some disorders such as NTBC treatment in type I tyrosinemia and cholic acid in bile acid synthetic disorders which allow avoiding transplantation in the majority of cases. Except for these 2 particular cases, the only medical treatment possible for cholestasis is a nonspecific treatment: ursodeoxycholic acid. The recent progresses in genetic diagnosis in cholestatic diseases could lead to a better comprehension of physiopathologic mechanisms and to the development of new therapeutic strategies such as liver cell transplantation or gene therapy.

References

1 Bernard O: Early diagnosis of neonatal cholestatic jaundice. Arch Pediatr 1998;5:1031–1035.
2 Setchell D, Dumaswala R, Colombo C, Ronchi M: Hepatic bile acid metabolism during early development revealed from the analysis of human fetal gallbladder bile. J Biol Chem 1988;263:16637–16644.
3 Jacquemin E: Development and physiopathology of biliary secretion. Arch Fr Pediatr 1992;49:741–748.
4 Chardot C, Carton M, Spire-Bendelac N, et al: Epidemiology of biliary atresia in France: a national study. J Hepatol 1999;31:1006–1013.
5 Chardot C, Carton M, Spire-Bendelac N, et al: Prognosis of biliary atresia in the era of liver transplantation: French national study from 1986 to 1996. Hepatology 1999;30:606–611.
6 Debray D, Parient D, Urvoas E, et al: Sclerosing cholangitis in children. J Pediatr 1994;12:49–56.
7 Amedee-Manesme O, Bernard O, Brunelle F, et al: Sclerosing cholangitis with neonatal onset. J Pediatr 1987;111:225–229.
8 Hadj-Rabia S, Baala L, Vabres P, et al: Claudin-1 gene mutations in neonatal sclerosing cholangitis associated with ichthyosis: a tight junction disease. Gastroenterology 2004;127:1386–1390.
9 Feldmeyer L, Huber M, Fellmann F, et al: Confirmation of the origin of the NISCH syndrome. Hum Mutat 2006;27:408–410.
10 Krawinkel MB: Parenteral nutrition-associated cholestasis – what do we know, what can we do? Eur J Pediatr Surg 2004;14:230–234.
11 Lang C, Meier Y, Stieger B, et al: Mutations and polymorphisms in the bile salt export pump and the multidrug resistance protein 3 associated with drug-induced liver injury. Pharmacogenet Genomics 2007;17:47–60.
12 Herzog D, Chessex P, Martin S, Alvarez F: Transcient cholestasis in new born infants with perinatal asphyxia. Can J Gastroenterol 2003;17:179–182.
13 Vajro P, Amelio A, Stagni A, et al: Cholestasis in new born infants with perinatal asphyxia. Acta Paediatr 1997;86:895–898.
14 Lykavieris P, Hadchouel M, Chardot C, Bernard O: Outcome of liver disease with Alagille syndrome: a study of 163 patients. Gut 2001;49:431–435.
15 Crosnier C, Driancourt C, Raynaud N, et al: Mutations in JAGGED1 gene are predominantly sporadic in Alagille syndrome. Gastroenterology 1999;116:1141–1148.
16 Teckman JH: Alpha1-antitrypsine deficiency in childhood. Semin Liver Dis 2007;27:274–281.
17 Regev A, Guaqueta C, Molina EG, et al: Does the heterozygous state of alpha1-antitrypsine deficiency have a role in chronic liver diseases? Interim results of a large case-control study. J Pediatr Gastroenterol Nutr 2006;43:S30–S35.
18 Hinds R, Hadchouel A, Shanmugham NP, et al: Variable involvement in siblings with PiZZ alpha-1-antitrypsine deficiency related liver disease. J Pediatr Gastroenterol Nutr 2006;43:136–138.
19 Lykavieris P, Bernard O, Hadchouel M: Neonatal cholestasis in childhood. Arch Dis Child 1996;75:67–70.
20 Englert C, Grabhorn E, Richter A, et al: Liver transplantation in children with progressive familial intrahepatic cholestasis. Transplantation 2007;84:1361–1363.
21 Bustorff-Silva J, Sbraggia Neto L, Olimpio H, et al: Partial internal biliary diversion through a cholecystojejunocolonic anastomosis – a novel surgical approach for patients with progressive familial intrahepatic cholestasis: a preliminary report. J Pediatr Surg 2007;42:1337–1340.
22 de Vree JM, Jacquemin E, Sturm E, et al: Mutation in the MDR3 gene cause progressive familial intrahepatic cholestasis. Proc Natl Acad Sci USA 1998;95:282–287.
23 Jung C, Driancourt C, Baussan C, et al: Prenatal molecular diagnosis of inherited cholestatis diseases. J Pediatr Gastroenterol Nutr 2007;44:453–458.
24 Russell DW, Setchell KDR: Bile acid biosynthesis. Biochemistry 1992;31:4737–4739.
25 Cheng JB, Jacquemin E, Gerhardt M, et al: Molecular genetics of 3beta-hydroxy-delta5-C27 steroid oxidoreductase deficiency in 16 patients with loss of bile acid synthesis and liver disease. J Clin Endocrinol Metab 2003;88:1833–1841.

26 Setchell KD, Heubi JE: Defects in bile acid biosynthesis – diagnosis and treatment. J Pediatr Gastroenterol Nutr 2006;43:17–22.
27 Yerushalmi B, Sokol RJ, Narkewicz MR, et al: Niemann-Pick disease type C in neonatal cholestasis at a North American center. J Pediatr Gastroenterol Nutr 2002;35:44–50.
28 Lee WS, Sokol RJ: Liver disease in mitochondrial disorders. Semin Liver Dis 2007;27: 259–273.
29 Lee WS, Sokol RJ: Mitochondrial hepatopathies: advance in genetics and pathogenesis. Hepatology 2007;45:1555–1565.
30 Bosch AM: Classical galactosemia revisited. J Inherit Metab Dis 2006;29:516–525.
31 McKiernan PJ: Nitisinone in the treatment of hereditary tyrosinemia type I. Drugs 2006; 66:743–750.
32 Van Spronsen FJ, Bijleveld CM, Van Maldegem BT, Wijburg FA: Hepatocellular carcinoma in hereditary tyrosinemia type I despite 2-(2 nitro-4-3 trifluoro- methylbenzoyl)-1, 3-cyclohexanedione treatment. J Pediatr Gastroenterol Nutr 2005;40:90–93.
33 Depreter M, Espeel M, Roels F: Human peroxisomal disorder. Microsc Res Tech 2003; 61:203–223.
34 de Lonlay P, Seta N, Barrot S, et al: A broad spectrum of clinical presentations in congenital disorders of glycosylation I: a series of 26 cases. J Med Genet 2001;38:14–19.
35 Jacquemin E, Lykavieris P, Chaoui N, et al: Transient neonatal cholestasis: origin and outcome. J Pediatr 1998;133:563–567.
36 Hermeziu B, Sanlaville D, Girard M, et al: Heterozygous bile salt export pump deficiency: a possible genetic predisposition to transient neonatal cholestasis. J Pediatr Gastroenterol Nutr 2006;42:114–116.

Annales Nestlé

Ann Nestlé [Engl] 2008;66:121–126
DOI: 10.1159/000147409

Familial Cholestatic Syndromes

Richard Thompson

Paediatric Hepatology, King's College London School of Medicine, London, UK

Key Words
Familial cholestatic syndromes · Alagille syndrome · Arthrogryposis, renal dysfunction and cholestasis syndrome · Familial intrahepatic cholestasis 1 deficiency · Bile salt export pump deficiency · Multidrug resistance protein 3 deficiency

Abstract
The term 'familial' is an unfortunate one. Although the definition includes 'hereditary', the inference is that it will usually have occurred in other family members. For many of the conditions described in this article this is often not the case, and for this reason, 'familial' conditions may be overlooked when reaching a diagnosis. Cholestasis is defined differently by clinicians, pathologists and biochemists. In addition, what is meant by cholestatic liver disease very often varies for paediatricians and adult hepatologists. However, the pathogenic mechanisms are increasingly similar. Biliary atresia, which is the most frequent cholestatic liver disease presenting to paediatricians, is strikingly different from most diseases as there appears to be no 'late-onset' equivalent and it is almost never familial. Several international collaborations have now been established in the hope of overcoming these hurdles (http://www.barcnetwork.org/, http://www.orpha.net/nestasso/EFBAR/, http://www.biliary-atresia.com/index_frameset_ebar.html). On a day-to-day basis, paediatric hepatologists are faced with a group of infants with jaundice in whom the cause is not readily apparent. In many ways, this has been worsened by the fact that we have known for a long time that a significant proportion will improve spontaneously, whereas others will do badly. In the first few months of life, we still have difficulty forecasting outcomes for individual patients. The underlying cause, at least in the group with a poor outcome, is now becoming apparent in an increasing number of cases. Most of the improvements in our unravelling of this group of children have come about as the result of advances in our understanding of the genetic aetiology. It has also become clear that genetic cholestatic liver disease is not restricted to paediatrics. The exact extent to which genetics contributes to 'late-onset' disease is only now being unravelled.

Genetics is not yet the first port of call in making a diagnosis in a cholestatic infant, though it may be soon [4]. The fact that cholestatic diseases are now being classified on the basis of their genetic cause makes it easier to identify phenotypic variations. These phenotypic differences improve both diagnosis and prognosis. They help us decide on the condition of a child, or at least suggest which gene or protein should be investigated. The phenotype extends to prognosis and particularly treatment outcomes, and a better understanding of these factors helps the clinician and the family alike. The major familial cholestatic syndromes are summarized in table 1.

KARGER

Fax +41 61 306 12 34
E-Mail karger@karger.ch
www.karger.com

© 2008 Nestec Ltd., Vevey/S. Karger AG, Basel
0517–8606/08/0663–0121$24.50/0

Accessible online at:
www.karger.com/ane

Richard Thompson
Institute of Liver Studies
King's College Hospital
Denmark Hill, London SE5 9RS (UK)
E-Mail richard.j.thompson@kcl.ac.uk

Table 1. The major familial cholestatic syndromes

Disease name	Aliases	Gene	Protein	Features
Alagille syndrome	arteriohepatic dysplasia	*JAG1*	Jagged 1	multisystem disorder, variable phenotype, heterozygous mutations in either gene
		NOTCH2	Notch 2	variable penetrance
ARC syndrome	Nezelof syndrome	*VPS33B*	VPS33B	multisystem disorder, mild cholestasis
FIC1 deficiency	Byler disease, PFIC1	*ATP8B1*	FIC1	multisystem disorder, wide range of severity
BSEP deficiency	Byler syndrome, PFIC2	*ABCB11*	BSEP	liver only affected, spectrum of severity
MDR3 deficiency	PFIC3	*ABCB4*	MDR3	liver only affected, wide range of severity

Alagille Syndrome

Alagille syndrome has always been a clinical diagnosis. In most cases, genetics would not be needed to diagnose an individual patient. Mutations were first identified in *JAGGED1,* which encodes a ligand in the Notch signalling pathway [5, 6]. Subsequently, in other patients, mutations have been identified in the gene encoding one of the Notch receptors, *NOTCH2* [7]. All in all, mutations have only been found on a single allele of the gene in question. One presumes that a loss of both alleles would be lethal, and certainly the mouse data would support this [8]. It is now clear that a genetic diagnosis can be arrived at in the vast majority of such individuals [9]. In many ways, this has only complicated things, particularly, as all published data concerning the frequency of different features and, more importantly, outcome data relate to patients diagnosed clinically. Although most patients have an identifiable genetic 'cause', it has long been known that family members can have similar, though milder, features. It is now clear that these relatives often share the same genetic abnormality. By no stretch of imagination could these individuals be said to have Alagille syndrome. This problem is all the greater when realising that in the general population, we have no idea of the frequency of mutations in the genes involved. Therefore, the diagnosis should probably remain a clinical one, until the true penetrance of mutations is established and the mechanisms that determine the phenotype are understood.

Arthrogryposis, Renal Dysfunction and Cholestasis Syndrome

Luckily, arthrogryposis, renal dysfunction and cholestasis syndrome (ARC) is rare. However, it does represent an important disease mechanism. In the same way as Alagille syndrome, it was described clinically. The phenotype as described was very severe, particularly in terms of the arthrogryposis, even though the liver disease was relatively mild. The gene mutated in the majority of cases has been identified as *VPS33B* [10]. Along with all the conditions described in the rest of this article, the mutations are recessive. It has long been known that many of the functions of the hepatocyte are highly polarised, with very different functions taking place at the basolateral and canalicular membranes (fig. 1). The protein encoded by *VPS33B* appears to be implicated in correctly sorting some proteins to the canalicular domain, and is not itself a trans-membrane transporter. It seems highly likely that other (possibly similar) phenotypes will be manifest if other proteins in this pathway are defective. However, as for the Alagille syndrome, patients have already been identified who do not have the complete phenotype [11]. This is important, as such patients would not have been classified as ARC previously, as they did not meet the clinical criteria. Again, this raises the, as yet unanswerable, question of how many patients with less severe phenotypes harbour mutations in these genes.

Familial Intrahepatic Cholestasis 1 Deficiency

Familial intrahepatic cholestasis 1, or FIC1, is the name generally applied to the protein encoded by *ATP8B1* [12]. This prosaic genetic nomenclature indicates that the protein is predicted to be P-type ATPase and is thus a relative of the Wilson disease gene. However, as discussed later, its function is probably quite different. FIC1 deficiency has been described as causing both benign recurrent intrahepatic cholestasis (BRIC) and progressive familial intrahepatic cholestasis (PFIC). In truth, it is evident that there are patients that fall between these 2 defined diseases, and that FIC1 deficiency is really a spectrum ranging from mild to severe liver disease [13]. This is clinically important as liver disease may progress, even in patients initially diagnosed with BRIC, often on the basis of a late presentation. Therefore, the term 'BRIC' is somewhat misleading and, indeed, may be falsely reassuring to both patients and their carers.

Many P-type ATPases are ion transporters, as is the case with the Wilson disease-associated protein. FIC1 on the other hand is thought to be one of several aminophospholipid flippases. The requirement for the maintenance of lipid asymmetry in biological membranes is clear, such that we probably have several of these proteins, expressed in a variety of tissues. The correct distribution of lipids between bilayers may well be essential for the sorting of proteins to the correct compartment. Equally, it is likely that the correct lipid composition of the plasma membrane is essential for the normal function of other protein therein. FIC1 deficiency not only manifests as cholestatic liver disease, but also with a highly variable set of other features. The most common are diarrhoea, hearing loss, renal tubular dysfunction and growth failure. Somewhat surprisingly, individuals can have severe manifestation of one aspect of the disease, with minimal features in another system. The multisystem nature of the disease is supported by the widespread expression of the *ATP8B1* gene [12]. In the liver, several proteins are not present, or present in significantly reduced quantities, in the canalicular membrane of patients with FIC1 deficiency. This is consistent with the hypothesis that abnormal membrane lipids are leading to abnormality of protein sorting similar in nature to ARC syndrome. Still, none of the proteins missing are known to be critical to bile formation or associated with cholestasis. In particular, immunohistochemical staining for the bile salt export pump (BSEP, itself discussed in more detail below) appears normal in FIC1 deficiency; however, recent data support another hypothesis [14]. Although largely based on a mouse model, this work does suggest that the FIC1 protein facilitates the movement of aminophospholipids from the outer to the inner leaflets of the plasma membrane [14], as was believed. The normal canalicular membrane needs to maintain a high degree of detergent resistance in order to prevent damage from the detergent effect of bile itself. The presence of excess aminophospholipids in the outer leaflet would reduce this detergent resistance. Using a short-term ex vivo bile acid infusion experiment, these investigators found evidence that the availability of aminophospholipids for extraction by bile acids is greatly increased in the knockout model. Furthermore, some of the canalicular ectoenzymes in the knockout livers are eluted

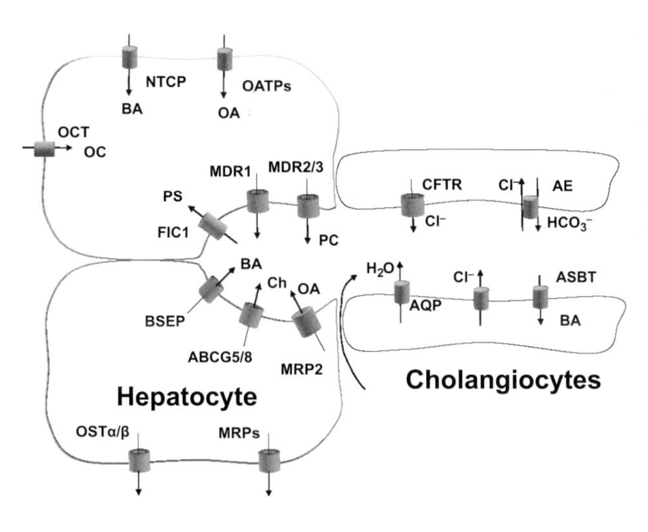

Fig. 1. The major transporters involved in bile formation in the hepatocyte and cholangiocyte membranes, many of which are now associated with familial cholestasis. ABCG5/8 = Heterodimeric cholesterol transporter; AE = anion exchanger; ASBT = apical sodium-dependent bile acid transporter; AQP = aquaporin; BA = bile acids; CFTR = cystic fibrosis transmembrane conductance regulator; Ch = cholesterol; FIC1 = familial intrahepatic cholestasis protein 1; MDR = multidrug resistance protein; MRP = multidrug resistance-associated protein; NTCP = sodium/taurocholate cotransporting polypeptide; OA = organic anions; OATP = organic anion-transporting poplypetide; OC = organic cations; OCT = organic cation transporter; OST = heterodimeric organic solute transporter; PS = phosphatidylserine.

in a bile salt-dependent fashion. These are some of the same enzymes previously shown to be absent from the human liver. This raises the possibility that these proteins have been removed from the canalicular membrane of human disease liver, instead of being subjected to a trafficking or targeting defect. This has not yet been proven in humans and it still does not account for cholestasis, as no transporter critical to bile formation has been shown to be absent. For these large proteins, it seems most likely that it is their function that is affected by the abnormal lipid composition of the canalicular membrane. The same may be the case in the other affected organs. In the ear, the kidney or the pancreas, it is clearly not the action of bile acids removing proteins that leads to the phenotype; there seems little doubt that the correct lipid composition of the membrane is critical to many functions. We are left with the additional complication of the highly variable phenotype. We know that there are several other aminophospholipid transporters in the human proteome. It seems likely that in FIC1 deficiency, the disease is only manifest where other proteins are not adequately compensating for the loss of FIC1 function. The extrahepatic manifestations of FIC1 deficiency limit the utility of liver transplantation. In particular, diarrhoea can get worse, and growth failure may not be impacted at all. The debilitating pruritus may be enough to justify the undertaking, but it cannot be regarded as a cure.

FIC1 deficiency was once called 'Byler disease', after the Amish family in which it was first described. Byler bile is the description of the canalicular contents seen in FIC1 deficiency on transmission electron microscopy. These unusual aggregates are not quite diagnostic of this condition, but are certainly highly suggestive. The knockout mouse develops a morphology indicative of Byler bile when fed cholic acid [14]. In the mouse, the appearances are highly suggestive of the granular components being formed from damaged microvilli, derived from the canalicular membrane. This loss of membrane surface area may, in itself, contribute to cholestasis. If the main mechanism by which the lack of FIC1 exerts its effect on the liver is by rendering the canalicular membrane susceptible to bile salt damage, it is surprising that the degree of morphological disruption seen on light microscopy is not greater. Yet again, it seems likely that even here, in the liver, the impact of the loss of FIC1 function is reduced by the presence of other lipid transporters and that a complete loss of aminophospholipid internalisation would probably lead to a significantly more severe liver disease.

BSEP Deficiency

The major bile salt transporter of the canalicular membrane, now referred to as the BSEP, is encoded by the gene *ABCB11.* In a fashion similar to that seen in FIC1 deficiency, patients have been identified with both mild (BRIC) [15] and severe (PFIC) [16, 17] phenotypes. The nomenclature is again unfortunate as there are undoubtedly patients all along the spectrum in between the 2 extremes. This is clinically extremely important as several so-called BRIC patients have features that suggest progressive liver disease, and the fact that a disease presents late, and may appear to remit, should not be taken as evidence that it will not cause later problems. The pathophysiology mechanisms leading to BSEP deficiency are somewhat easier to understand. A complete, or partial, failure of bile acid transport, at the canalicular membrane, is going to have an obvious effect on hepatocellular function. It is clear that the hepatocyte disarray is much greater than that seen in FIC1 deficiency, often showing considerable giant cell transformation in infancy. BSEP appears not to be expressed outside the liver, and therefore, the clinical feature can entirely be accounted for by a failure of bile salt transport at the canalicular membrane. The clinical manifestations are those of severe cholestasis, though, as bilirubin is transported quite separately from bile salts, the degree of jaundice can markedly underestimate the degree of cholestasis. Liver transplantation is an excellent form of treatment for BSEP deficiency.

In children, hepatocellular carcinoma (HCC) is extremely rare. Cholangiocarcinoma is even rarer. On the other hand, hepatoblastoma is the commonest hepatocyte-derived malignancy, along with the much rarer fibrolamellar HCC. Both of these malignancies occur against the background of a normal liver, not in the context of chronic liver disease. In children, HCC is seen with some specific diseases, notably, classical tyrosinaemia and, to a lesser extent, glycogen storage diseases. Ten young children with HCC and BSEP deficiency were reported following a search for children with HCC against the background of a severe neonatal hepatitis picture [18]. The exact risk for each patient is difficult to assess, particularly as many patients are transplanted before developing this complication. In a subsequent study, 2 children with cholangiocarcinomata, again presenting against the background of a neonatal hepatitis, were found to have BSEP deficiency [19]. A subsequent analysis of 128 children with mutation-proven, severe BSEP deficiency found that 19 had had the one or the other malignancy [17]. The risk appears to be much greater if the individual has 2 protein-truncating mutations (38 vs. 10% in other genotypes). Many patients had had early transplantation, without developing malignancy. In the absence of transplantation, the risk must be considerably higher. All these patients had clinically severe disease; there was no apparent correlation between disease severity and risk of malignancy. Considering that other children with persistent cholestasis do not seem to develop malignancy, one is forced to question the mechanism by which the neoplastic change occurs. The obvious candidate of damage induced by the retained bile salts is thrown into doubt by several of the above observations. It is only possible to speculate as to the true mechanism. However, it is certainly possible that BSEP is normally transporting low levels of something other than bile salts, which is caused to accumulate in its absence, or perhaps, BSEP has some other function entirely, the complete absence of which leads to malignancy. Whatever the mechanism, the risk is real and must be taken into account when considering all modes of treatment, other than transplantation, be they pharmacological, surgical or genetic. All will presumably leave a risk of malignancy, requiring very close monitoring.

Multidrug Resistance Protein 3 Deficiency

In the course of human evolution, we have become extremely efficient at extracting fat from our diet. In much of the world, where calories are in abundance, we are paying the price. However, in order to be so good at extracting fat from our diet we have evolved the ability to synthesise highly detergent bile acids. Bile acids, by their very nature, are toxic. When retained in the liver, they lead to severe disease; as seen in BSEP deficiency. However, after transportation into bile they achieve millimolar concentrations. Therefore, bile itself has the potential to cause severe damage to the biliary tree. Indeed, whatever triggers sclerosing cholangitis, or biliary atresia, bile in the form of bile acids does much of the damage. Humans and many mammals have had to evolve mechanisms to minimise the toxic effects of bile acids. A major mechanism by which we do this is by enabling the formation of mixed micelles. These are composed of bile acids and other lipids, most notably phosphatidylcholine (PC). The entry of lipids, particularly PC, into bile to form micelles is closely coupled to bile acid flux. The data relating to FIC1 deficiency, discussed above, suggest that bile acids can extract lipids from the canalicular membrane in a rather non-specific fashion if they are made available. Normally, this does not happen, as most of the membrane is detergent resistant. Instead, PC seems to be extracted in a highly specific fashion. We now recognise multidrug resistance protein 3 (MDR3) as being essential for the entry of PC into bile [20]. The availability of PC in the outer leaflet of the canalicular membrane appears to be tightly controlled by MDR3. Therefore, even a minor loss of MDR3 function would be expected to change the composition of bile. Indeed, a whole range of phenotypes have been described associated with reduced MDR3 function, including propensity of gallstone formation [21, 22]. Patients with only one defective copy can manifest symptoms under certain circumstances, for example during pregnancy [23, 24], though they are otherwise well. The severe end of the spectrum, PFIC, seems relatively rare. This condition is readily distinguished from FIC1 and BSEP deficiencies as it is associated with elevated levels of circulating γ-glutamyl transferase. However, as MDR3 mutations are increasingly sought, late-onset MDR3-related disease, including small duct sclerosing cholangitis, AMA-negative primary biliary cirrhosis and even cryptogenic cirrhosis are being identified. Whether MDR3 really plays a major role in cholesterol cholelithiasis remains to be seen. However, in pedigrees with multiple affected individuals, particularly if the stones are intrahepatic, mutations within this gene are not uncommon [25].

Conclusions

In the last 10 years, our understanding of the molecular mechanisms involved in bile formation and cholestasis has improved dramatically. Analysis of families segregating different forms of liver disease has played a significant part in these advances. In addition, we can now see that some late-onset conditions have, in some cases, a genetic cause, and in others, a genetic susceptibility. The full extent to which late-onset liver diseases are actually milder versions of these conditions remains to be seen; we have probably only scratched the surface so far. Within paediatrics, it is now essential to convert this understanding into better outcomes for patients. In the United States, a multi-centre collaboration is seeking to do just that [26]. Much of the published retrospective data include patients we would now consider to be poorly characterised. With our greatly improved techniques and knowledge, we should now be able to make diagnoses more quickly, understand the disease processes better and plan treatment and trials in light of this knowledge.

References

1 Biliary Atresia Research Consortium. http://www.barcnetwork.org/.
2 European Federation of Biliary Atresia Research. http://www.orpha.net/nestasso/EFBAR/.
3 European Biliary Atresia Registry. http://www.biliary-atresia.com/index_frameset_ebar.html.
4 Liu C, Aronow BJ, Jegga AG, et al: Novel resequencing chip customized to diagnose mutations in patients with inherited syndromes of intrahepatic cholestasis. Gastroenterology 2007;132:119–126.
5 Oda T, Elkahloun AG, Pike BL, et al: Mutations in the human Jagged1 gene are responsible for Alagille syndrome. Nat Genet 1997;16:235–242.

6 Li L, Krantz ID, Deng Y, et al: Alagille syndrome is caused by mutations in human Jagged1, which encodes a ligand for Notch1. Nat Genet 1997;16:243–251.
7 McDaniell R, Warthen DM, Sanchez-Lara PA, et al: NOTCH2 mutations cause Alagille syndrome, a heterogeneous disorder of the notch signaling pathway. Am J Hum Genet 2006;79:169–173.
8 Xue Y, Gao X, Lindsell CE, et al: Embryonic lethality and vascular defects in mice lacking the Notch ligand Jagged1. Hum Mol Genet 1999;8:723–730.
9 Warthen DM, Moore EC, Kamath BM, et al: Jagged1 (JAG1) mutations in Alagille syndrome: increasing the mutation detection rate. Hum Mutat 2006;27:436–443.
10 Gissen P, Johnson CA, Morgan NV, et al: Mutations in VPS33B, encoding a regulator of SNARE-dependent membrane fusion, cause arthrogryposis-renal dysfunction-cholestasis (ARC) syndrome. Nat Genet 2004;36:400–404.
11 Bull LN, Mahmoodi V, Baker AJ, et al: VPS33B mutation with ichthyosis, cholestasis, and renal dysfunction but without arthrogryposis: incomplete ARC syndrome phenotype. J Pediatr 2006;148:269–271.
12 Bull LN, van Eijk MJ, Pawlikowska L, et al: A gene encoding a P-type ATPase mutated in two forms of hereditary cholestasis. Nat Genet 1998;18:219–224.
13 van Mil SW, Klomp LW, Bull LN, et al: FIC1 disease: a spectrum of intrahepatic cholestatic disorders. Semin Liver Dis 2001;21:535–544.
14 Paulusma CC, Groen A, Kunne C, et al: Atp8b1 deficiency in mice reduces resistance of the canalicular membrane to hydrophobic bile salts and impairs bile salt transport. Hepatology 2006;44:195–204.
15 van Mil SW, van der Woerd WL, van der Brugge G, et al: Benign recurrent intrahepatic cholestasis type 2 is caused by mutations in ABCB11. Gastroenterology 2004;127:379–384.
16 Strautnieks SS, Bull LN, Knisely AS, et al: A gene encoding a liver-specific ABC transporter is mutated in progressive familial intrahepatic cholestasis. Nat Genet 1998;20: 233–238.
17 Strautnieks SS, Byrne JA, Pawlikowska L, et al: Severe bile salt export pump deficiency: 82 different ABCB11 mutations in 109 families. Gastroenterology 2008;134:1203–1214.
18 Knisely AS, Strautnieks SS, Meier Y, et al: Hepatocellular carcinoma in ten children under five years old with bile salt export pump deficiency. Hepatology 2006;44:478–486.
19 Scheimann AO, Strautnieks SS, Knisely AS, et al: Mutations in bile salt export pump (ABCB11) in two children with progressive familial intrahepatic cholestasis and cholangiocarcinoma. J Pediatr 2007;150:556–559.
20 de Vree JM, Jacquemin E, Sturm E, et al: Mutations in the MDR3 gene cause progressive familial intrahepatic cholestasis. Proc Natl Acad Sci USA 1998;95:282–287.
21 Rosmorduc O, Hermelin B, Poupon R: MDR3 gene defect in adults with symptomatic intrahepatic and gallbladder cholesterol cholelithiasis. Gastroenterology 2001;120: 1459–1467.
22 Jacquemin E, De Vree JM, Cresteil D, et al: The wide spectrum of multidrug resistance 3 deficiency: from neonatal cholestasis to cirrhosis of adulthood. Gastroenterology 2001;120:1448–1458.
23 Dixon PH, Weerasekera N, Linton KJ, et al: Heterozygous MDR3 missense mutation associated with intrahepatic cholestasis of pregnancy: evidence for a defect in protein trafficking. Hum Mol Genet 2000;9:1209–1217.
24 Jacquemin E, Cresteil D, Manouvrier S, et al: Heterozygous non-sense mutation of the MDR3 gene in familial intrahepatic cholestasis of pregnancy. Lancet 1999;353:210–211.
25 Rosmorduc O, Poupon R: Low phospholipid associated cholelithiasis: association with mutation in the MDR3/ABCB4 gene. Orphanet J Rare Dis 2007;2:29.
26 Cholestatic Liver Disease Consortium. http://rarediseasesnetwork.epi.usf.edu/clic/index.htm.

Annales Nestlé

Ann Nestlé [Engl] 2008;66:127–135
DOI: 10.1159/000147410

Treatments in Chronic Cholestasis in Children

Fernando Alvarez

CHU Sainte-Justine, University of Montreal, Montreal, Qué., Canada

Key Words
Chronic cholestasis · Ursodeoxycholic acid · Rifampicin · Ion exchange resins · ω-3 fatty acids · N-acetyl cysteine · Opioid antagonist

Abstract
Few specific treatments for children with chronic cholestasis are available. Most therapy strategies relieve bile component retention or palliate some of the consequences of chronic cholestasis. Ursodeoxycholic acid is the most frequently used pharmacological agent in children with chronic cholestasis. This bile acid is administered at dosages between 10 and 30 mg/kg/day to patients with cystic fibrosis, inborn errors of bile acid metabolism, progressive familial intrahepatic cholestasis, sclerosing cholangitis, biliary atresia, Alagille syndrome, or those receiving total parenteral nutrition. Ursodeoxycholic acid mainly increases bile flow and has a membrane-stabilizing effect, reducing the toxicity of more hydrophobic bile acids. Rifampicin, an antibiotic, at dosages between 10 and 20 mg/kg/day is very efficient in relieving pruritus. Similar effects are obtained using nonabsorbable ion exchange resins. In addition, these molecules decrease the serum cholesterol levels contributing to reduce xanthomas. Replacement of some deficiencies created by total parenteral nutrition by administration of essential fatty acids or cysteine can prevent or contribute to improve the associated liver disorders. In some cholestatic diseases, surgical procedures can help to relieve the obstacle to the bile flow, as it is the case for portoenterostomy in patients with biliary atresia. In cases of intrahepatic cholestasis, a clinical and biochemical improvement can be recorded after bile diversion or other procedure (ileum exclusion) limiting the absorption of bile acids by the intestine. In the future, the association of these different pharmacological agents, increasing the bile flow, protecting cell membranes, or restoring nutritional deficiencies, could contribute to an improvement in quality of life in children with chronic cholestasis and eventually delay the need of a more drastic therapy such as liver transplantation. Advances in gene therapy and hepatocyte transplantation could also be of great help; however, many years of intense research are still necessary before even a pilot study using one of these therapies can be considered on liver diseases resulting in chronic cholestasis.

Chronic cholestasis in children is the consequence of a large variety of causes, and very few of them have a specific treatment. In most cases, medical or surgical therapies have been developed to prevent or treat complications secondary to bile component retention. Existing treatments are mostly supportive, trying to reduce the accumulation of bile acids in the organism and its consequences: progressive liver fibrosis, pruritus, hyperlipidemia and fatigue.

Reduced quantities of bile acids in the lumen of the intestine are responsible for fat malabsorption. Steatorrhea can become a cause of malnutrition and liposoluble vitamin deficiency in chronic cholestasis. Some therapies

KARGER

Fax +41 61 306 12 34
E-Mail karger@karger.ch
www.karger.com

0517–8606/08/0663–0127$24.50/0

Accessible online at:
www.karger.com/ane

Prof. Fernando Alvarez, MD
Division of Gastroenterology, Hepatology and Nutrition
CHU Sainte-Justine, University of Montreal
3175, Cote Sainte-Catherine road, Montreal, Qué. H3T 1C5 (Canada)
E-Mail fernando.alvarez@umontreal.ca

Table 1. Available treatments for chronic cholestasis in children

Treatment	Indication	Contraindication	Side effects	Dosage
UDCA	influence on the pathogenesis of PFIC, CF, TPN; 'pruritus'	obstruction of bile ducts (e.g., failure of portoenterostomy in BA)	diarrhea	20–30 mg/kg/day
Rifampicin	'pruritus'	mycobacterium infection[1]		10–20 mg/kg/day
Nonabsorbable ion exchange resins	'pruritus' hypercholesterolemia	intestinal stenosis or subocclusion	constipation hyperchloremic acidosis	8–16 g orally daily divided in 2–3 times (increased progressively from 2 g orally daily)
Opioid antagonists	'pruritus'	–	withdrawal reactions	?
ω-3 fatty acids	TPN-induced liver disease	–	–	1 g/kg/day (increased progressively from 0.2 mg/kg/day)
NAC	TPN-induced liver disease	–	–	70–135 mg/kg/day (increased progressively from 20 mg/kg/day)

Associations of some of these drugs are usually required. BA = Biliary atresia.

described below, aiming to avoid the enterohepatic recirculation of bile acids, can aggravate this situation.

Pharmacological agents such as ursodeoxycholic acid (UDCA) and rifampicin improve choleresis by enhancing hepatocyte excretion of bile acids. Nonabsorbable ion exchange resins bind bile acids in the lumen of the intestine, decreasing its enterohepatic circulation. All these drugs increase choleresis and diminish pruritus and levels of cholesterol. Opioid antagonists have been proposed to treat pruritus; however, their limited availability, as well as their side effects, restricted their use in pediatrics (table 1).

Surgical interventions can be curative, as the Kasai intervention in some patients with biliary atresia, or palliative as the partial biliary diversion and the ilial exclusion in patients with Alagille syndrome or progressive familial intrahepatic cholestasis (PFIC). The latter could improve pruritus, decrease cholesterol retention and prevent evolution to cirrhosis.

Ursodeoxycholic Acid

UDCA (3α,7β-dihydroxy-5β-cholan-24-oic acid) is present in small quantities in human bile, up to 3%, and is the result of the 7β epimerization of chenodeoxycholic acid by colonic bacteria [1].

The β rather than the α hydroxy group at the 7th position gives UDCA a higher hydrophilicity when compared with chenodeoxycholic acid, its precursor. Thus, because of less hydrophobicity, UDCA is poor at micelle formation. In addition, it is poorly absorbed in the proximal intestine [1].

Mechanisms of Action

- Replacement of more hydrophobic bile acids at the circulating pool and at cell membranes. After 6 months of treatment at 10–12 mg/kg/day, UDCA represents 40–50% of the bile acid pool [2]. Because of their detergent capabilities, more hydrophobic bile acids are toxic for cell membranes, causing hepatocellular damage and an increase in cholestasis. UDCA has a membrane-stabilizing effect, reducing disruption of cholesterol-rich membranes [3].
- UDCA, but not its conjugated form taurodeoxycholate, decreases the toxicity of lipophilic bile acids on the function of the electron transport chain in a concentration-dependent form (up to 100 μmol/l), but increases bile acid-induced mitochondrial toxicity at higher concentrations [4].
- Interference in the ileum with the absorption of more toxic bile acids [2].
- UDCA is reabsorbed by the biliary epithelium in a protonated form and it is secreted again into bile (cholehepatic shunt) producing a hypercholeretic effect.

The protons absorbed lead to the formation of bicarbonate that is secreted and enrich the bile in this component [2].

- UDCA increases the bile salt-independent flow [1, 2].
- UDCA may stimulate transporter expression at the canalicular hepatocyte surface [5].
- A reduction in human leukocyte antigen class I expression at the hepatocyte surface has been reported [6].
- UDCA also suppresses interferon-γ-mediated induction of human leukocyte antigen class II expression via the glucocorticoid receptor-mediated pathway [7].

UDCA is responsible for very few and transitory side effects, such as diarrhea and skin reactions more probably due to drug adjuvants than to the active substance. However, it should be avoided or carefully administered to patients with an obstructive bile duct disease. In experimental animals with a ligation of the main bile duct, UDCA can aggravate bile infarcts [8]. In children with biliary atresia and unsuccessful Kasai intervention, UDCA can precipitate a liver failure.

UDCA is the most frequent drug used in children with chronic cholestasis. In several diseases, the benefit of the long-term administration of UDCA has not been proven beyond any doubt, as is the case for cystic fibrosis (CF). In other cases, the administration of the drug improves liver tests, but not the final outcome, as in patients with sclerosing cholangitis. In PFIC, it appears to stop the progression of the disease in some children and, associated with cholic acid, it is the treatment of choice in patients with inborn errors of the bile acid metabolism. In children with Alagille syndrome or biliary atresia, UDCA is mainly used to reduce symptoms such as pruritus.

Cystic Fibrosis

After 2 months of UDCA therapy, the presence of this bile acid represents between 25 and 42% of the pool, at the expense of cholic and chenodeoxycholic acids; these differences are dose dependent [9]. From these studies, it was concluded that the recommended dosage of UDCA is 20 mg/kg/day or greater [9].

UDCA stimulates the biliary secretory capacity in livers of CF patients, as determined by hepatobiliary scintigraphy [10]. Several pilot studies have shown that UDCA is responsible for an improvement in biochemical tests, mainly a decrease in serum levels of aminotransferases (ALT and AST) and γ-glutamyl transferase (GGT) [11]. In addition, liver inflammation and/or bile duct proliferation were improved after 2 years of UDCA therapy in control biopsies. UDCA administration also improves the nutritional state of young adults with CF and, in children, ameliorates essential fatty acids and retinol status [12–14]. However, because of poor UDCA activity in micelle formation it did not affect steatorrhea [13]. If UDCA modifies the natural history of liver diseases in CF patients, it still remains to be studied in a large randomized prospective study. Encouraging results were recently reported on UDCA-induced arrest or even reversion of liver ultrasound lesions observed in patients with CF, in a long-term study [15].

Total Parenteral Nutrition

Fasting associated with total parenteral nutrition (TPN) leads to bile stasis related to lack of stimulation of the bile acid-dependent and -independent bile flow. In a model of TPN-induced cholestasis, the intravenous administration of UDCA improved bile flow and reduced bilirubin levels [16]. Similar encouraging results were recorded in a pilot study of children with intractable diarrhea depending on TPN, but tolerating UDCA at the dosage of 30 mg/kg/day in 3 daily doses [17].

In very low birth weight infants with TPN-associated cholestasis, UDCA at doses of 10–30 mg/kg/day reduces the duration and intensity of cholestasis [18]. In most of these patients, intestinal complications, including partial resections of the bowel, preclude the standard use of UDCA. Eventually, a very fractionated daily dosage of the medication can be well tolerated, avoiding diarrhea. Unfortunately, the UDCA intravenous form is not commercially available.

Inborn Errors of Bile Acid Metabolism

Two main forms of bile acid synthesis defect are responsible for chronic cholestasis in children: the 3-oxo-Δ4-steroid 5β-reductase deficiency and the 3β-hydrosteroid-Δ5-oxireductase/isomerase deficiency. Hepatotoxicity is probably due to the accumulation of bile acid precursors and the lack of primary bile acids. To reduce the synthesis of toxic molecules, the activity of cholesterol 7α hydroxylase, the rate-limiting enzyme in endogenous bile acid synthesis, must be inhibited.

Most patients respond only partially to UDCA treatment alone; association of cholic acid (250 mg/day) is therefore indicated. The administration of chenodeoxycholic and cholic acids has also been proposed in these patients. The latter treatment can lead to a faster improvement in the liver injury [19].

Progressive Familial Intrahepatic Cholestasis

UDCA is a valuable initial treatment for patients with PFIC when administered orally at doses between 20 and

30 mg/kg/day. Similar improvement was observed no matter the PFIC type, meaning patients with normal (PFIC types 1 and 2) or increased levels (PFIC type 3) of serum GGT. In patients with normal GGT, an improvement in parameters of cholestasis was observed in 61% of cases and in 71% of those with type 3 PFIC [20]. The duration of the disease prior to the beginning of the UDCA treatment could influence these results; early diagnosis and initiation of UDCA therapy could further improve the final outcome. In some patients, the improvement, even if complete, is only transitory, and the cholestasis reappears some years after the beginning of UDCA.

In patients with less deleterious mutations in genes responsible for types 1 or 2 of PFIC, a benign recurrent intrahepatic cholestasis is observed. In benign recurrent intrahepatic cholestasis patients, UDCA treatment fails in preventing a cholestatic episode, but could improve some of the symptoms (e.g., pruritus) [21].

Sclerosing Cholangitis

An initial pilot study of UDCA in patients with well-developed sclerosing cholangitis showed an improvement in liver tests. Later, a statistically significant difference in the serum levels of ALT/AST/GGT was observed between UDCA and placebo-treated patients with sclerosing cholangitis during a study of 3 years of follow-up [22]. An improvement in pruritus and fatigue was also observed, but the difference was not significant. Unfortunately, more recent results in a randomized, double-blind study comparing UDCA (13–15 mg/kg/day) with placebo showed no differences in treatment failure (progression of the disease, death or liver transplantation). This study confirmed an improvement in liver tests, but concluded that UDCA did not offer clinical benefits to patients with sclerosing cholangitis [23]. Thus, low dosages of UDCA apparently do not modify the progression of this disease. A very recently published study showed that, on the contrary, high doses of UDCA were associated with an improvement in survival and a trend toward stability/improvement in the histological stage in a relatively small group of patients with sclerosing cholangitis [24].

Despite these results, new trials could be proposed using high dosages of UDCA very early in the evolution of sclerosing cholangitis, and particularly in patients with small duct disease. When the disease affects the main bile ducts (as in most cases), probably, the disturbance in the bile flow can contribute irreversibly to the aggravation of the liver disease. The larger experience in the use of UDCA in chronic cholestatic diseases was obtained in adult patients with primary biliary cirrhosis, a severe form of intrahepatic cholangiopathy [25]. Different groups showed controversial results with UDCA therapy, partially explained by the different time in the evolution of the disease at the starting of treatment. The dose of UDCA administered also appears to play a role in the influence of this medication on the final outcome. This vast experience should be considered in planning new trials in patients with sclerosing cholangitis.

Biliary Atresia

An early preliminary study using UDCA after hepatic portoenterostomy showed that this drug was effective in patients with a good postoperative bile drainage, resulting in lower total bile acid levels and better weight gain [26]. Long-term administration of UDCA significantly improves the final outcome after Kasai portoenterostomy, more patients cleared jaundice and survived with their native liver. In children without recovery of a good bile flow after portoenterostomy, UDCA administration can lead to faster development of liver injury, and eventually, precipitates a liver failure [27].

Alagille Syndrome

Few reports are available on the use of UDCA in patients with Alagille syndrome. Improvement in the jaundice and pruritus was found, as well as a decrease in circulating lipid levels and a decrease in xanthomas [28]. No controlled study is available; however, UDCA is widely prescribed to these patients. The influence of this bile acid in the natural history of the disease is still unknown.

Rifampicin

Rifampicin decreases the bile acid concentration in hepatocytes, by competing with its uptake. Furthermore, this antibiotic induces microsomal enzymes that promote the 6α-hydroxylation and subsequent 6α-glucuronidation of toxic bile acid.

Initial clinical experience using this antibiotic for the treatment of pruritus was given in adults with a primary biliary cirrhosis, showing a significant relief from pruritus in a majority of patients [29]. In children with chronic cholestasis, a double-blind crossover study showed the efficacy of rifampicin in alleviating pruritus during a period of up to 6 months [30]. Subsequently, 2 studies on pediatric patients with refractory pruritus treated by rifampicin confirmed those initial results [31, 32]. No improvement in biochemical features of cholestasis was recorded in most treated children with different causes of chronic cholestasis.

The recommended dosage of rifampicin is 10–20 mg/kg/day in 2 daily doses. Few side effects were reported. However, rifampicin is an enzymatic inducer of microsomal enzymes. Several forms of cytochrome P450 isoenzyme activity are increased by rifampicin administration; therefore, the rate of metabolism of several drugs can be accelerated.

It was proposed that UDCA and rifampicin have complementary effects that may justify a combination of both agents in the treatment of patients with cholestatic diseases [33].

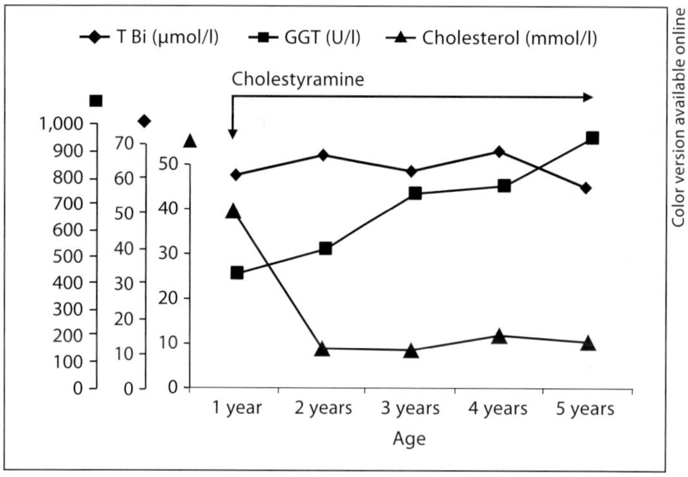

Fig. 1. In this boy with Alagille syndrome, cholestyramine was administered by a nasogastric tube, indicated for enteral feeding. Dramatic decrease in serum cholesterol levels and shrinking of xanthomas was observed. Pruritus improved with the association of rifampicin with the treatment. No modifications in biochemical parameters of cholestasis were recorded.

Nonabsorbable Ion Exchange Resins

These molecules are not absorbable from the gastrointestinal tract and release chloride and bind bile acids in the lumen of the intestine, diminishing their enterohepatic recirculation. Nonabsorbable ion exchange resins augment cholesterol excretion via enhanced conversion to bile acids. These drugs can decrease the bile acid pool by approximately 40%. Trihydroxy bile acid dissociates rapidly from these molecules and can be absorbed in the ileum.

Cholestyramine (orange-flavored granules) has been used for some decades and has been proven to be effective and safe. However, palatability is poor, limiting the tolerability to this drug. Therefore, compliance is erratic in the best of cases. When nasogastric tubes are indicated for enteral feeding, the administration of cholestyramine through this pathway has been shown to be well tolerated and successful in decreasing serum cholesterol levels and improving pruritus (fig. 1).

In children, cholestyramine can be started at a dosage of 2–4 g twice daily and then increased to 8–16 g daily in 2 or 3 divided doses. Cholestyramine binds other acids or negatively charged substances, which explains most of its interaction with many drugs.

Colestipol in granules or tablets has not been used frequently in children. Indications and precautions in its use are similar to those described for cholestyramine.

Colesevelam hydrochloride (in the form of a nonabsorbable hydrogel or tablet) is probably the best tolerated of these drugs, but unfortunately, it is not available everywhere [34]. This drug has enhanced the specificity, greater affinity and higher capacity for binding bile acids compared with the 2 other nonabsorbable ion exchange resins mentioned above.

Nonabsorbable ion exchange resins can interfere with the intestinal absorption of other drugs, like UDCA. This particular problem should be considered when treating a patient with chronic cholestasis. In addition, the time of administration should be well established to allow a maximal capture of bile acids and to avoid interaction with other drugs including fat-soluble vitamins. Other drugs should be given 1 or 4–6 h after cholestyramine.

Main side effects are constipation and hyperchloremic acidosis due to the large quantities of chloride released in the gastrointestinal lumen and absorbed instead of bicarbonate. The latter can be particularly severe in patients with Alagille syndrome, frequently showing previous renal problems.

Opioid Antagonists

Naloxone and nalmefene are the first 2 opioid antagonists tested in adults with primary biliary cirrhosis, attempting to relieve pruritus [35, 36]. The use of these substances was based on the possible role of the central nervous system in the pruritus observed in patients with cholestasis. Enkephalin class substances (endogenous opioids) may be potential mediators in the involvement of the nervous system.

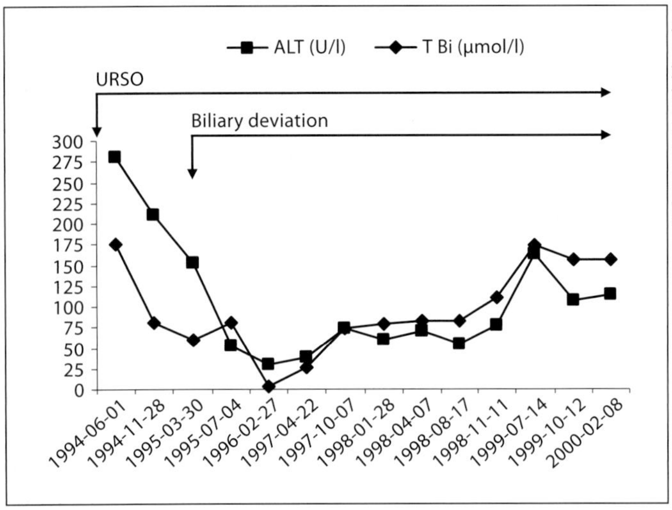

Color version available online

Fig. 2. In this girl with PFIC (low GGT), a partial biliary deviation was carried out. An almost complete normalization of biochemical liver tests was recorded. Relapse of symptoms and signs of cholestasis were observed 2–3 years after surgery. Hepatobiliary scintigraphy showed that the bile flow was almost exclusively directed to the stoma bag. This case showed that the liver disease progressed despite bile diversion and UDCA treatment.

A placebo-controlled single-blinded trial of naloxone proved that this medication reduced the scratching activity in cholestatic patients. The main problems with this drug were the need of intravenous perfusions due to its very short half-life and a possible opiate withdrawal syndrome at the end of the perfusion [35].

Nalmefene can be administered orally (but this form is not available everywhere). Improvement in the perception of pruritus was reported in most treated patients because of its longer duration of action when compared with naloxone. This medication can be associated with severe withdrawal symptoms, which is apparently dependent on the dosage used. Marked exarcebation of pruritus when the drug was suddenly discontinued was also reported [36].

Naltrexone can also be administered orally. In a randomized trial of naltrexone versus placebo, a significant decrease in daytime and nighttime itching was reported. Opiate withdrawal syndrome was observed in half of the patients receiving naltroxone [37].

No series on the use of opioid antagonists in children with chronic cholestasis has been published. Therefore, it is impossible to conclude on its indication in the pediatric population. From adult experiences, these drugs are difficult to administer and it is hard to avoid side effects when discontinued.

ω-3 Fatty Acids

Liver disease associated with TPN in children with intestinal failure can lead to cirrhosis and liver failure. In some patients, when UDCA is absorbed, an improvement in liver tests has been recorded. More spectacular results were obtained by replacing soy oils in fat emulsions with fish oils. Children receiving a solution enriched in ω-3 fatty acids showed a dramatic improvement in the liver disease [38].

Recently, a 4-year-old boy followed at our institution had a resection of most of his small intestine, because of a volvulus. This child developed a severe liver disease on TPN and was enrolled on the waiting list for a liver transplant. Parenteral fish oil was started (Omegaven), and 3 months later, he was removed from the waiting list, and 6 months later, showed normal serum levels of conjugated bilirubin [V. Marchand, pers. commun.].

N-Acetyl Cysteine

Liver disease in the long-term TPN population is the consequence of a variety of factors. Oxidative stress appears to play a major role in the etiology and in the persistence and aggravation of cholestasis. Cellular concentrations of glutathione is an essential defense against this harmful process. Cysteine is an important precursor of intracellular glutathione; however, low levels of cysteine are found in currently used aminoacid solution.

N-acetyl cysteine (NAC) can be used as a precursor of cysteine. When NAC was added to the parenteral nutrition solution, at dosages of 70–135 mg/kg/day, a normalization or marked decrease in serum-conjugated bilirubin levels was recorded [39]. This improvement in liver cholestasis was associated with a normalization of glutathione in red blood cells, suggesting that the cellular concentration of this antioxidant molecule played a major role in the decrease in the liver injury.

Surgical Procedures

Biliary Diversion and Ileal Exclusion

More than 30 years ago, Alagille and Odièvre, at Bicêtre Hospital in France, described the efficacy of biliary drainage by cholecystostomy in patients with PFIC and Alagille syndrome. Unfortunately, because of local complications on the skin around the drain, this type of external bile drainage could not be kept for a long time [40].

In the 80s, a technique of partial biliary diversion was developed, using 10–15 cm of jejunum interposed between the gallbladder and the skin. This procedure was permanent and allowed the partial deviation of the bile flow to an external stoma bag for years. A clinical and biochemical improvement was reported in patients with Alagille syndrome [41]. In children with PFIC, the partial biliary diversion resulted in an improvement in growth, relief of pruritus and correction of biochemical anomalies of cholestasis [42, 43]. In some cases, the dramatic improvement was transitory, followed by a relapse of the cholestasis and the requirement of liver transplantation after 4–5 years of the initial bile deviation (personal observations) (fig. 2). In other cases, the complete improvement was only obtained if UDCA was given as a coadjuvant therapy.

A technical variant was later reported, in which the appendix vermiformis was used as a conduit between the gallbladder and the skin, with very good results [44].

In a recent publication, another way of obtaining a partial deviation of the bile flow was described. In 3 patients with Alagille syndrome, 15% of the terminal ileum was excluded using a stapled division and ileocecal anastomosis. The rationale of the procedure is to avoid the site of maximal absorption of bile acids in the bowel. A decrease in cholesterol levels, an improvement in pruritus and a reduction in xanthomes sizes were observed [45].

All of these surgical procedures should be avoided in patients that have already developed a cirrhosis. Important bleeding from neo-varices at sites of anastomosis is a very frequent complication. In addition, in patients with advanced liver disease, the benefits of such procedures are not demonstrated.

Hepaticoportoenterostomy

The surgical intervention described by Kasai in the 1950s became the first and only procedure able to restore the bile flow in patients with biliary atresia.

Normalization of serum bilirubin, within 3 months of portoenterostomy, has been found to indicate a good long-term prognosis. This occurs in around 50–60% of operated infants, with a better outcome when the intervention has been carried out early in life [46]. Other factors at the time of the portoenterostomy can modify the final outcome such as the degree of the liver fibrosis and the characteristics of the extrahepatic remnant. The prognosis of the Kasai intervention in a patient with polysplenia malformation syndrome associated with biliary atresia has been worse in some centers and similar to biliary atresia without malformations in others [47]. In the postoperatory period, the development of cholangitis can also worsen the prognosis.

Because of the presence of inflammatory infiltrate in the liver of these patients, it was proposed that the use of anti-inflammatory drugs could arrest the progression of the disease. Unfortunately, several recent publications of pilot and double-blind randomized studies showed that the use of high doses of steroids after Kasai intervention did not increase survival of the native liver [48, 49].

Ten-year survival is between 30 and 54% in different centers around the world; around 25% at 20 years, and 10% at 30 years [50–53]. All patients develop a cirrhosis, with the associated complications of portal hypertension: gastrointestinal bleeding, hypersplenism and hepatopulmonary diseases.

Liver transplantation has improved the overall survival of children with biliary atresia and failure of the Kasai intervention. Currently, the success of this therapy is responsible for a survival rate of 90% [47].

Perspectives

Eventually, 2 future therapies could definitely cure some inherited diseases responsible for chronic cholestasis: gene therapy and/or hepatocyte transplantation. In the case of gene therapy, after initial years of hope, disappointing results in most trials and serious side effects relented its progression and further development. In the case of the liver, it is not known how many cells should express a specific gene to avoid the development of symptoms and signs of a particular disease and impede its progression. Many problems need to be solved before we can even think of a trial concerning a cholestatic liver disease.

Hepatocyte transplantation has already been attempted in some human beings. Partial correction of liver-inherited diseases was observed in animal models. Normal hepatocytes have an advantage over the repopulation of the liver against cells carrying a mutated and possibly lethal gene. Correction of the PFIC type 3 in a mouse model was reported and stayed stable for a long time [54]. This therapy is confronted with the availability of normal hepatocytes, the need of immunosuppressive therapy and the question on the fate of remaining mutated cells. The risk of tumors developing in the long-term follow-up represents a considerable concern.

The use of ω-3 fatty acid cholestasis of different origins should be explored. Deficiency in essential fatty acids has been reported in patients with cholestasis of different etiologies, e.g., Alagille syndrome and CF. This feature is most probably a consequence of severe steatorrhea. Extraintestinal pathways of administration have been proposed, but without much success. Intravenous, periodic administration could be indicated in some cases.

Oxidative stress is almost constantly associated with cholestasis. It can be hypothesized that in these children, the retention of bile components, the malabsorption responsible for malnutrition and deficiency of essential fatty acids and oligoelements lead to malformation of different cellular mechanisms of protection. In the latter, the deficiency in glutathione can be included. NAC administration could be of great help in several cholestatic processes, as an adjuvant therapy.

Future trials should test the potential benefit of ω-3 fatty acids and NAC in children with chronic cholestasis. Both of these therapies show very few side effects, being well tolerated in children.

Many of the drugs described above could be associated in the treatment of chronic cholestasis in order to diminish the liver injury and/or to relieve harmful symptoms of these disorders. Drugs with different mechanisms of action can be associated with an adequate nutritional support, individualizing the therapy according to the etiology of the cholestasis and the current status of a particular child.

References

1 Heuman DM: Hepatoprotective properties of ursodeoxycholic acid. Gastroenterology 1993;104:1865–1870.
2 Beuers U, Boyer JL, Paumgartner G: Ursodeoxycholic acid in cholestasis: potential mechanisms of action and therapeutic applications. Hepatology 1998;28:1449–1453.
3 Heuman DM, Bajaj R: Ursodeoxycholate conjugates protect against disruption of cholesterol-rich membranes by bile salts. Gastroenterology 1994;106:1333–1341.
4 Krahenbuhl S, Fischer S, Talos C, Reichen J: Ursodeoxycholate protects oxidative mitochondrial metabolism from bile acid toxicity: dose-response study in isolated rat liver mitochondria. Hepatology 1994;20:1595–1601.
5 Fickert P, Zollner G, Fuchsbichler A, et al: Effects of ursodeoxycholic and cholic acid feeding on hepatocellular transporter expression in mouse liver. Gastroenterology 2001;121:170–183.
6 Terasaki S, Nakanuma Y, Ogino H, et al: Hepatocellular and biliary expression of HLA antigens in primary biliary cirrhosis before and after ursodeoxycholic acid therapy. Am J Gastroenterol 1991;86:1194–1199.
7 Tanaka H, Makino Y, Miura T, et al: Ligand-independent activation of the glucocorticoid receptor by ursodeoxycholic acid. Repression of IFN-gamma-induced MHC class II gene expression via a glucocorticoid receptor-dependent pathway. J Immunol 1996; 156:1601–1608.
8 Fickert P, Zollner G, Fuchsbichler A, et al: Ursodeoxycholic acid aggravates bile infarcts in bile duct-ligated and Mdr2 knockout mice via disruption of cholangioles. Gastroenterology 2002;123:1238–1251.
9 Colombo C, Crosignani A, Assaisso M, et al: Ursodeoxycholic acid therapy in cystic fibrosis-associated liver disease: a dose-response study. Hepatology 1992;16:924–930.
10 Colombo C, Castellani MR, Balistreri WF, et al: Scintigraphic documentation of an improvement in hepatobiliary excretory function after treatment with ursodeoxycholic acid in patients with cystic fibrosis and associated liver disease. Hepatology 1992;15: 677–684.
11 Colombo C, Setchell KD, Podda M, et al: Effects of ursodeoxycholic acid therapy for liver disease associated with cystic fibrosis. J Pediatr 1990;117:482–489.
12 Lindblad A, Glaumann H, Strandvik B: A two-year prospective study of the effect of ursodeoxycholic acid on urinary bile acid excretion and liver morphology in cystic fibrosis-associated liver disease. Hepatology 1998;27:166–174.
13 Cotting J, Lentze MJ, Reichen J: Effects of ursodeoxycholic acid treatment on nutrition and liver function in patients with cystic fibrosis and longstanding cholestasis. Gut 1990;31:918–921.
14 Lepage G, Paradis K, Lacaille F, et al: Ursodeoxycholic acid improves the hepatic metabolism of essential fatty acids and retinol in children with cystic fibrosis. J Pediatr 1997;130:52–58.
15 Nousia-Arvanitakis S, Fotoulaki M, Economou H, et al: Long-term prospective study of the effect of ursodeoxycholic acid on cystic fibrosis-related liver disease. J Clin Gastroenterol 2001;32:324–328.
16 Duerksen DR, Van Aerde JE, Gramlich L, et al: Intravenous ursodeoxycholic acid reduces cholestasis in parenterally fed newborn piglets. Gastroenterology 1996;111:1111–1117.
17 Spagnuolo MI, Iorio R, Vegnente A, Guarino A: Ursodeoxycholic acid for treatment of cholestasis in children on long-term total parenteral nutrition: a pilot study. Gastroenterology 1996;111:716–719.
18 Chen CY, Tsao PN, Chen HL, et al: Ursodeoxycholic acid (UDCA) therapy in very-low-birth-weight infants with parenteral nutrition-associated cholestasis. J Pediatr 2004; 145:317–321.
19 Clayton PT, Mills KA, Johnson AW, et al: Delta 4-3-oxosteroid 5 beta-reductase deficiency: failure of ursodeoxycholic acid treatment and response to chenodeoxycholic acid plus cholic acid. Gut 1996;38:623–628.
20 Jacquemin E, Hermans D, Myara A, et al: Ursodeoxycholic acid therapy in pediatric patients with progressive familial intrahepatic cholestasis. Hepatology 1997;25:519–523.
21 Crosignani A, Podda M, Bertolini E, et al: Failure of ursodeoxycholic acid to prevent a cholestatic episode in a patient with benign recurrent intrahepatic cholestasis: a study of bile acid metabolism. Hepatology 1991;13: 1076–1083.

22 Stiehl A, Walker S, Stiehl L, et al: Effect of ursodeoxycholic acid on liver and bile duct disease in primary sclerosing cholangitis. A 3-year pilot study with a placebo-controlled study period. J Hepatol 1994;20:57–64.
23 Lindor KD: Ursodiol for primary sclerosing cholangitis. Mayo Primary Sclerosing Cholangitis-Ursodeoxycholic Acid Study Group. N Engl J Med 1997;336:691–695.
24 Cullen SN, Rust C, Fleming K, et al: High dose ursodeoxycholic acid for the treatment of primary sclerosing cholangitis is safe and effective. J Hepatol 2008;48:792–800.
25 Corpechot C, Carrat F, Bahr A, et al: The effect of ursodeoxycholic acid therapy on the natural course of primary biliary cirrhosis. Gastroenterology 2005;128:297–303.
26 Nittono H, Tokita A, Hayashi M, et al: Ursodeoxycholic acid in biliary atresia. Lancet 1988;1:528.
27 Stringer MD, Davison SM, Rajwal SR, McClean P: Kasai portoenterostomy: 12-year experience with a novel adjuvant therapy regimen. J Pediatr Surg 2007;42:1324–1328.
28 Krawinkel MB, Santer R, Oldigs HD: Ursodesoxycholic acid: effect on xanthomas in Alagille-Watson syndrome. J Pediatr Gastroenterol Nutr 1994;19:476–477.
29 Bachs L, Parés A, Elena M, et al: Comparison of rifampicin with phenobarbitone for treatment of pruritus in biliary cirrhosis. Lancet 1989;1:574–576.
30 Cynamon HA, Andres JM, Iafrate RP: Rifampin relieves pruritus in children with cholestatic liver disease. Gastroenterology 1990;98:1013–1016.
31 Gregorio GV, Ball CS, Mowat AP, Mieli-Vergani G: Effect of rifampicin in the treatment of pruritus in hepatic cholestasis. Arch Dis Child 1993;69:141–143.
32 Yerushalmi B, Sokol RJ, Narkewicz MR, et al: Use of rifampin for severe pruritus in children with chronic cholestasis. J Pediatr Gastroenterol Nutr 1999;29:442–447.
33 Marschall HU, Wagner M, Zollner G, et al: Complementary stimulation of hepatobiliary transport and detoxification systems by rifampicin and ursodeoxycholic acid in humans. Gastroenterology 2005;129:476–485.
34 Aldridge MA, Ito MK: Colesevelam hydrochloride: a novel bile acid-binding resin. Ann Pharmacother 2001;35:898–907.
35 Bergasa NV, Talbot TL, Alling DW, et al: A controlled trial of naloxone infusions for the pruritus of chronic cholestasis. Gastroenterology 1992;102:544–549.
36 Bergasa NV, Schmitt JM, Talbot TL, et al: Open-label trial of oral nalmefene therapy for the pruritus of cholestasis. Hepatology 1998;27:679–684.
37 Wolfhagen FH, Sternieri E, Hop WC, et al: Oral naltrexone treatment for cholestatic pruritus: a double-blind, placebo-controlled study. Gastroenterology 1997;113:1264–1269.
38 Gura KM, Duggan CP, Collier SB, et al: Reversal of parenteral nutrition-associated liver disease in two infants with short bowel syndrome using parenteral fish oil: implications for future management. Pediatrics 2006;118:e197–e201.
39 Mager DR, Marcon M, Wales P, Pencharz PB: Use of N-acetyl cysteine for the treatment of parenteral nutrition-induced liver disease in children receiving home parenteral nutrition. J Pediatr Gastroenterol Nutr 2008;46:220–223.
40 Alagille D, Odievre M: Les cholestases de l'enfant. Maladies du foie et des voies biliaires chez l'enfant. Paris, Flammarion, 1978.
41 Emerick KM, Whitington PF: Partial external biliary diversion for intractable pruritus and xanthomas in Alagille syndrome. Hepatology 2002;35:1501–1506.
42 Melter M, Rodeck B, Kardorff R, et al: Progressive familial intrahepatic cholestasis: partial biliary diversion normalizes serum lipids and improves growth in noncirrhotic patients. Am J Gastroenterol 2000;95:3522–3528.
43 Kurbegov AC, Setchell KD, Haas JE, et al: Biliary diversion for progressive familial intrahepatic cholestasis: improved liver morphology and bile acid profile. Gastroenterology 2003;125:1227–1234.
44 Gauderer MW, Boyle JT: Cholecystoappendicostomy in a child with Alagille syndrome. J Pediatr Surg 1997;32:166–167.
45 Modi BP, Suh MY, Jonas MM, et al: Ileal exclusion for refractory symptomatic cholestasis in Alagille syndrome. J Pediatr Surg 2007;42:800–805.
46 Ohhama Y, Shinkai M, Fujita S, et al: Early prediction of long-term survival and the timing of liver transplantation after the Kasai operation. J Pediatr Surg 2000;35:1031–1034.
47 Chardot C, Serinet MO: Prognosis of biliary atresia: what can be further improved? J Pediatr 2006;148:432–435.
48 Davenport M, Stringer MD, Tizzard SA, et al: Randomized, double-blind, placebo-controlled trial of corticosteroids after Kasai portoenterostomy for biliary atresia. Hepatology 2007;46:1821–1827.
49 Petersen C, Harder D, Melter M, et al: Postoperative high-dose steroids do not improve mid-term survival with native liver in biliary atresia. Am J Gastroenterol 2008;103:712–719.
50 McKiernan PJ, Baker AJ, Kelly DA: The frequency and outcome of biliary atresia in the UK and Ireland. Lancet 2000;355:25–29.
51 Chardot C, Carton M, Spire-Bendelac N, et al: Prognosis of biliary atresia in the era of liver transplantation: French national study from 1986 to 1996. Hepatology 1999;30:606–611.
52 Shneider BL, Brown MB, Haber B, et al: A multicenter study of the outcome of biliary atresia in the United States, 1997 to 2000. J Pediatr 2006;148:467–474.
53 Schreiber RA, Barker CC, Roberts EA, et al: Canadian Pediatric Hepatology Research Group. Biliary atresia: the Canadian experience. J Pediatr 2007;151:659–665.
54 De Vree JM, Ottenhoff R, Bosma PJ, et al: Correction of liver disease by hepatocyte transplantation in a mouse model of progressive familial intrahepatic cholestasis. Gastroenterology 2000;119:1720–1730.

Annales Nestlé

Ann Nestlé [Engl] 2008;66:137–147
DOI: 10.1159/000147411

Nutritional Management of Cholestatic Syndromes in Childhood

Piotr Socha

Department of Gastroenterology, Hepatology and Immunology, The Children's Memorial Health Institute, Warsaw, Poland

Key Words
Liver disease · Lipid-soluble vitamins · Vitamin E · Malnutrition · Enteral nutrition · Parenteral nutrition · Liver failure

Abstract
Cholestatic liver disease causes severe risk of malnutrition which includes protein-energy malnutrition and specific nutritional deficiencies. The nutritional status can be assessed based on anthropometric measurements, which can be misleadinq because of ascitis and peripheral edema. Biochemical determinations of lipid-soluble vitamin status are important to evaluate requirements. Based on nutritional status assessment, nutritional therapy should be planned according to a well-defined schedule. The basic principle of nutritional management is to correct the nutritional status as well as to reduce the risk of nutritional deficiencies. Children with cholestasis usually need extra energy supply that can be obtained by increasing energy density of feeds or addition of glucose polymers and lipids. For catch-up growth, usually, protein intake should be increased. Lipid-soluble vitamin supplementation deserves special attention and it is not easy to correct poor vitamin E status. For some children, parenteral administration of vitamin K is needed. Since recently, a water-soluble vitamin E (d-α-tocopheryl polyethylene glycol 1000 succinate) given by oral route is used with a good therapeutic effect. As the liver disease progresses to liver failure in many chronic cholestatic diseases, nutritional therapy can often be regarded as 'bridging' for liver transplantation to improve prognosis. Thus, invasive nutritional support is justified in severe liver disease which usually includes nocturnal nasogastric tube feeding, or even parenteral nutrition.

Introduction

Requirements of specific nutrients for healthy infants and children are widely discussed and recommendations are updated every few years. There are still many controversies concerning some nutrients. Recently, vitamin K supplementation in infancy was a matter of debate. Ijland et al. [1] questioned the safety of oral vitamin K supplementation in a daily dose of 25 μg in a healthy population as bleeding occurred in 6 breastfed infants in the population studied. Apparently, 5 out of 6 bleeding infants were cholestatic children with biliary atresia. Thus, cholestasis caused the risk of vitamin K deficiency and the results do not necessarily point to the need to change recommendations for healthy infants. One should be aware that these recommendations do not apply to cholestasis which is a specific risk group. Cholestatic liver disease should be recognized early and specific treatment started as early as possible. Many cholestatic liver diseases progress to

KARGER

Fax +41 61 306 12 34
E-Mail karger@karger.ch
www.karger.com

0517–8606/08/0663–0137$24.50/0

Accessible online at:
www.karger.com/ane

Prof. Piotr Socha
Department of Gastroenterology, Hepatology and Immunology
The Children's Memorial Health Institute, Al. Dzieci Polskich 20
PL–04-730 Warsaw (Poland)
E-Mail p.socha@czd.pl

liver insufficiency and require liver transplantation. Nutritional therapy seems to be one of the priorities and can be regarded as a 'bridging' for liver transplantation. Nutritional status is an important prognostic factor, and children with better nutritional status have fewer complications and lower mortality at liver transplantation [2]. This is the reason why we recently elaborated and published guidelines on nutrition of infants with cholestatic liver disease [3].

We have almost forgotten diseases related to specific nutrient deficits. Recently, Samonte et al. [4] described a young girl who underwent liver transplantation and had a long battle with complications presenting as end-stage renal disease and liver failure. She developed classical oral signs of scurvy which were confused with cyclosporine toxicity, skin changes suggested vasculitis and bone aches were regarded to be related to renal osteodystrophy or corticosteroid-induced osteoporosis. Finally, it appeared that the disease was caused by vitamin C deficiency. In the editorial to this publication, we indicate that there are still situations where we can find basic diseases, caused by deficiency of one nutritional component [5]. Severe liver disease with cholestasis is a very good example of these nutritional problems.

In this chapter, causes of malnutrition, specific nutrient requirements and a nutritional approach to children with cholestatic liver disease are presented and discussed.

Causes of Malnutrition

Diminished bile flow leading to decreased intraluminal bile acid concentration seems to be the major pathomechanism responsible for malnutrition. Cholestasis leads to a significant decrease in lipid absorption and long-chain triglycerides require bile acids for utilization. Lipids significantly contribute to energy uptake, and thus, their malabsorption may cause a negative energy balance. High requirements of other nutrients like protein and carbohydrate are also documented. Many studies show that absorption and utilization of lipids and lipid-soluble vitamins is a process of several stages: dispersion in lipid emulsion, solubilization into mixed bile salt micelles, movement across the unstirred water layer adjacent to the microvilli, cellular uptake by intestinal mucosal cells, incorporation into chylomicrons, and secretion into the lymph. Absorption of some vitamins in cholestasis may be severely reduced, like vitamin E or β-carotene; other vitamins are better utilized, and high-dose supplementation can efficiently balance poor absorption. There are several other indicators of deficiency risk that should be evaluated: low caloric intake, unbalanced diet with low fat and vegetable consumption, increased oxidative status due to recurrent infections and some other chronic disease conditions complicating liver disease. For these high-risk groups, special attention is needed.

Increased energy expenditure was also documented in cholestasis and it can increase up to 40% or more for body weight in malnutrition but it is normal if calculated for age [6, 7]. Anorexia is a common problem of advanced liver disease and it can be attributed to organomegaly or ascitis. Portal hypertension with naturally occurring shunts may have central effects of unidentified toxins. As important growth hormones like insulin-like growth factor 1 and its binding proteins are produced by the liver in response to circulating growth hormone, cholestasis and portal hypertension may lead to abnormal insulin-like growth factor 1 axis response. These abnormalities cannot be corrected by hyperalimentation [8].

Can We Use a Standard Approach to All Cholestatic Diseases?

In general, severe cholestasis progressing to end-stage liver disease causes significant malabsorption and requires intensive nutritional management. Still, it is difficult to describe a standard approach. Usually, listing for liver transplantation is an indication for nutritional therapy according to standardized protocols. However, some cholestatic diseases progress slowly to liver insufficiency or may not require liver transplantation. Progressive familial intrahepatic cholestasis (PFIC) can be treated by a surgical procedure described as partial biliary diversion. This treatment is able to stop progression of liver damage, but vitamin or β-carotene malabsorption is not corrected. This disease requires special nutritional attention as vitamin E levels are extremely low in these patients and they are not directly related to the degree of cholestasis. In this disease, severe steatorrhea is often documented, which is not related to pancreatic insufficiency [9]. High requirements of vitamin E supplements are also observed in children operated for biliary atresia, but they correspond well with the degree of cholestasis.

Another metabolic problem discussed in cholestasis is a high cholesterol level observed in Alagille syndrome. Some liver centers use only low cholesterol diet to treat this abnormality, other centers use pharmacotherapy to lower cholesterol levels. The recent publication comparing intima media thickness as an indicator of atherogenesis in patients with PFIC (presenting with low cholesterol levels) and Alagille syndrome shows that patients with PFIC are at higher risk for cardiovascular disorders involving atherosclerosis. Intima media thickness and wall stiffness were increased in patients with PFIC but not in patients with Alagille syndrome. Total cholesterol, low-density lipid cholesterol, high-density lipid cholesterol and lipoprotein X were remarkably increased in patients with Alagille syndrome, whereas in patients with PFIC, an increase in triglyceride and a decrease in high-density lipid cholesterol were the prominent findings [10]. Thus, a nutritional approach should not primarily aim at decreasing cholesterol levels in Alagille syndrome.

Assessment of the nutritional status may also cause some problems. Short stature is a typical feature of PFIC and it cannot be corrected by nutritional support. That is why height is not a good indicator of nutritional status in PFIC (fig. 1).

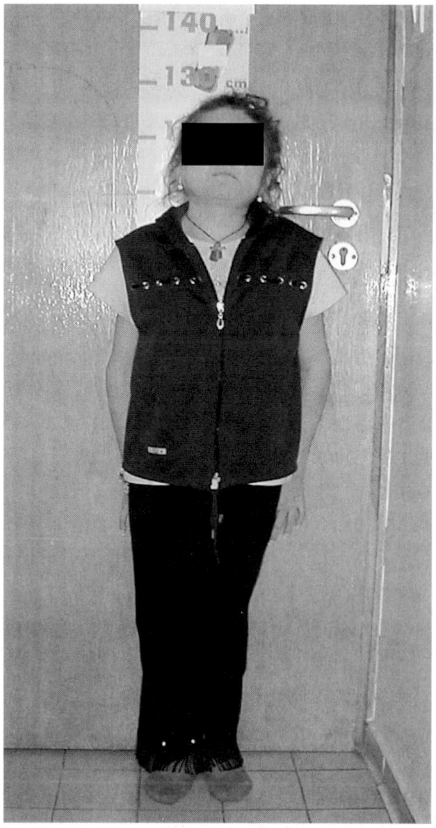

Color version available online

Fig. 1. Short stature – a 14-year-old girl with PFIC.

Diagnosis of Nutritional Deficiencies

Protein-energy malnutrition can be easily recognized if special nutritional support is not introduced from the early beginning of cholestasis. Children may present with thin limbs and a prominent abdomen. Body weight is not regarded as a good indicator of nutritional status as it is affected by fluid balance abnormalities [11, 12]. However, if ascitis is efficiently managed with diuretics, changes of body weight may be used for the evaluation of nutritional status. Other anthropometric parameters may be used to assess the nutritional status like mid upper arm circumference and triceps skin fold thickness. Height may be affected if malnutrition is prolonged. That is why the assessment of nutritional status may be complicated, and it should also take into account the specific liver disease.

Specific nutrient deficits cannot be easily recognized and they should be prevented as early as possible. However, the clinical symptoms of nutrient deficiencies still occur in clinical practice – scurvy or bleeding are only examples. That is why it is extremely important to detect any signs of malnutrition very early. As pointed out in the guidelines, all children with cholestatic liver disease should have a full nutritional review with an intervention and follow-up plan documented in their case records [3]. Energy, protein, carbohydrate and lipid intake as well as vitamin supplements should be recorded. Dieticians must be involved in nutrition assessment and planning. Still, careful dietary monitoring may not be sufficient to avoid malnutrition and significant body composition changes. Some deficiencies may not accompany protein-energy malnutrition and can be precociously detected only by biochemical measurements. This raises the following questions: should lipid-soluble vitamins be evaluated in high-risk group patients? Secondly, should we routinely supplement vitamins and increase energy intake in these high-risk patients? The answer to the first question is positive. We can precisely describe high-risk groups where periodic vitamin evaluation could be beneficial in terms of early diagnosis of deficiency. The answer to the second question is more difficult. Although vitamin K and E supplementation is regarded as safe, excess of vitamins A and D in some circumstances may be detrimental and may cause severe complications.

Jaundiced patients develop osteoporosis more frequently than nonjaundiced patients. Vitamin D defi-

Table 1. Deficiency monitoring – vitamins and minerals

Nutritional element	Clinical signs of deficiency	Signs of toxicity	Biochemical monitoring
Vitamin A	usually not observed – dry skin, xerophthalmia and night blindness	liver fibrosis, hypercalcemia, pseudotumor cerebri and painful bone lesions	serum retinol/RBP ≥0.8 serum retinol 250–800 ng/ml
Vitamin D	osteopenia, bone fractures, hypocalcemia, metaphyseal changes, hypophosphatemia, muscle hypotonia and rickets	hypercalcemia and pseudotumor cerebri	25-OH-D serum levels >25 ng/ml
Vitamin E	neuropathy, edema, anemia, skin lesions	not documented in cholestatic children; extremely high doses may affect neutrophyl chemotaxis and protein carboxylation vitamin K dependent; safety of supplementation questioned in adults in respect of cardiovascular disease	vitamin E/total lipids ≥0.6 mg/g serum α-tocopherol 3.8–16 mg/l
Vitamin K	hemorrhage	not documented	prothrombin time PIVKA II <3 ng/ml
Water-soluble vitamins	usually do not occur; anemia may be related to folic acid and vitamin B_6 deficiency, neuropathy to B_1 and B_{12} deficiency, and scurvy to vitamin C deficiency	not observed with normal doses	usually not performed; in specific high-risk groups, vitamin C can be monitored
Iron	anemia, behavioral changes	serum ferritin, iron and hemoglobin are not very reliable	
Minerals: calcium selenium zinc phosphate	osteoporosis, osteopenia, bone fractures, growth failure, skin lesions, anorexia, neutropenia	not observed with normal doses; still, selenium given in high doses can be toxic	serum calcium concentration and urinary calcium/creatinine excretion as lab routines, serum selenium, zinc concentration in selected labs

RBP = Retinol-binding protein.

ciency seems to be responsible. Bone-mineral deficiency can be detected earlier by means of bone mineral density measurement (noninvasive method) than by measuring serum Ca, P and Mg levels in these patients (table 1) [13].

Energy and Carbohydrate Intake

As energy requirements increase significantly in chronic cholestasis, energy-dense feeds can be used to increase caloric intake. In clinical practice, some liver units use concentrated infant formulae for cholestatic infants where energy density may increase up to 50%. Carbohydrates and proteins may be added to normal feeds. Carbohydrate is the major source of dietary energy contributing about two thirds of the non-protein energy. Short-chain polymers are currently used in nutritional support as their osmotic load is not high enough to cause diarrhea. Starch may also be used but it can cause bloating and diarrhea if not digested in the small intestine. The patients should be monitored for side effects when short-chain polymers are increased subsequently during a few days. If there are significant symptoms of intolerance, the carbohydrate dose should not be further increased. Even if carbohydrates are used as the main source of energy, lipids can also contribute to the higher energy requirements. Still, carbohydrates are usually better accepted by the patients as they have better taste than lipids or protein.

Calculation of carbohydrates added to the usual feeds should be based on estimated energy requirements, which increase significantly in end-stage liver disease and in biliary atresia with severe cholestasis.

Water and Electrolytes

Fluid requirement is normal for actual weight if restriction is not needed because of ascitis or edema. Sodium should not be supplemented in high amounts to correct hyponatremia as it can cause fluid retention. In infancy, sodium intake of 1 mmol/kg/day and normal potassium of about 2 mmol/kg/day are usually appropriate [3]. It is difficult to find the appropriate balance between fluid restriction and high-energy demand. That is the reason why energy-dense feeds should be used.

Protein

Children with normal growth and weight usually require normal protein intake. Maintenance needs do not appear to be very different from those of healthy children. However, advanced cholestatic liver disease with malnutrition should be managed with intensive nutritional therapy and a higher protein intake to support high rates of catch-up growth. A 10% protein/energy ratio used to rehabilitate malnourished children is generally sufficient to ensure rapid catch-up growth if only energy needs are covered [14]. The specific needs in cholestasis are not clearly described. Infants with severe cholestatic liver disease seem to require a protein intake of around 2–3 g/kg/day. The requirements are lower in cholestasis in childhood as it is the case for healthy children and infants. Infections often observed in biliary atresia (like cholangitis episodes) may further increase energy and protein requirements. In children, proteolysis increases markedly during infections and a negative protein balance may occur [15]. Protein restriction can be considered only if encephalopathy is present – that is in case of liver failure and of portosystemic shunts related to portal hypertension. Hyperammonemia does not justify protein restriction, in absence of encephalopathy.

A polymeric diet is systematically used for infants and children with cholestatic liver disease. Protein hydrolysates may be considered in enteral nutrition or temporarily in severe malnutrition. The taste of feeds should also be considered as an important factor as poor palatability may further decrease energy intake. Thus, hydrolysates can be used only in very specific clinical situations.

Recently, branched-chain amino acids were tested in animal models and in clinical settings of biliary atresia [16, 17]. They improved weight gain, muscle mass, nitrogen balance and also led to increased total body potassium, mid upper arm circumference and subscapular skinfold thickness in cholestatic children.

The recent guidelines proposed an ideal product which would include protein as 3 g/kg/day of whey proteins, being approximately 2.6 g/100 ml reconstituted formula, enriched in branched-chain amino acid to 10%, treating hyperammonemia instead of reducing protein intake [3].

Lipids

The dietary supply and metabolism of lipids in early childhood are of major importance for growth, body composition and child development. The choices of dietary lipid during the first years of life are of great practical importance for growth and development not only in healthy infants and children, but even more in children with hepatic disorders. Lipids are the major source of energy supplied by human milk. The supply of dietary lipids is also important for providing essential lipid-soluble vitamins and polyunsaturated fatty acids (PUFAs) [18].

Lipids as Energy Source

Lipid absorption is markedly decreased in cholestasis which leads to decreased energy intake. Thus, it is important to balance the energy losses with extra energy supply. Carbohydrates may increase energy density of feeds to some extent but they are not sufficient to cover all energy needs. Lipids are less palatable, but other features of this macronutrient make it a valuable dietary supplement: high energy density, low osmolarity and content of essential PUFAs. Steatorrhea may limit lipid use in nutritional support, even though in a child with steatorrhea, growth may improve if lipids, given in higher amounts, increase fat intake [19]. Medium-chain triglycerides (MCTs) can be optionally used as a lipid supplement or as an MCT-enriched formula. MCTs do not provide the same energy balance as long-chain triglycerides (LCTs) but they are successfully used in the treatment of fat malabsorption because they have a high water solubility and are rapidly cleaved by lipases [20]. However, because of the shorter chain length of their fatty acids, their energy content (per gram of fat) is about 16% lower than that of LCTs. MCTs are rapidly oxidized and have a high thermogenic effect. They reach the liver directly via the portal flow without need for formation of mixed micelles but they are also ketogenic [21]. Larger amounts of dietary MCTs are metabolized in several tissues by carnitine-dependent mechanism and may increase the need for carnitine [22]. One may estimate the proportion of 30–50% of total lipids as MCTs as the optimal for nutritional management in cholestasis [23, 24]. Still, it is difficult to specify the ideal dietary fat content and ratio of MCTs to LCTs. Limited data point to better fat solubilization and growth of cholestatic infants fed with 30 or 70% MCTs against a 50/50% mixture of MCTs/LCTs [25]. Essential fatty acid deficiency was described with the use of very high MCT content in the diet which was not sufficiently supplemented with PUFAs [23]. Most of the infant formulae with MCTs have an MCT/LCT ratio of about 1/1 and are supplemented with essential fatty acids. The MCT-rich formulae for children may contain higher amounts of MCTs (75 to >80% of lipids; e.g., Caprilon and Portagen) even though they are supplemented with essential fatty acids. Special attention is needed if pure MCT oil is used as a dietary supplement, and in this situation, a detailed dietary assessment is required. PUFA-rich vegetable oils should also be used to support adequate intake of essential fatty acids. Lipid intake and MCT ratio should be titrated against optimal weight gain and growth and intolerance of nutrients. Lipids should be used to increase energy density and a proportion at least similar to that for healthy age-matched children (from 30 to 50%) seems to be reasonable [3].

Polyunsaturated Fatty Acids

Long-chain PUFAs (LCPs, PUFAs with a carbon chain length >18), such as arachidonic (AA) and docosahexaenoic acid (DHA), are important for early human growth and development of membrane-rich tissues such as the brain and retina [26]. PUFAs are also precursors of eicosanoids with important biological roles as mediators of immune and vascular functions and platelet aggregation, making PUFA deficiency (especially from the n-6 series) a concern. The classical essential fatty acids linoleic acid (18:2n-6) and α-linolenic acid (18:3n-3) must be delivered with the diet and then are elongated in the liver and in the brain to obtain LCPs [18]. Breastfed infants receive appreciable amounts of preformed AA and DHA with human milk lipids [27]. In contrast to infants fed with human milk, those fed conventional milk formulae based on vegetable oils do not receive appreciable amounts of LCPs with their diet and depend on the utilization of body stores or endogenous synthesis from essential fatty acid precursors for LCP provision for growing tissues. Koletzko et al. [28] estimated conversion rates of linoleic acid with a stable isotope technique and found that the contribution of AA synthesis to the total plasma AA pool is only about 6% per day. Still, to draw any conclusions on the benefits of LCP supply in infancy, strong evidence from randomized clinical trials is needed. A Cochrane review of 2004 reviewed publications on LCP supplementation in term infants up to 2001 which included studies on visual acuity as well as on cognitive function and psychomotor development [29]. Different methods were applied to measure the functional effects of supplements which causes difficulties for drawing conclusions. The authors concluded that a beneficial effect of LCP supply on information processing is possible, but larger studies over longer periods are suggested to further investigate this issue. In a critical review of the available publications, Uauy et al. [30] pointed out that some studies that did not find advantages of LCPs either used low concentrations of DHA or did not include an assessment of compliance.

Recent publications which were not included in the Cochrane review studied later LCP supply in infants after weaning from breastfeeding in the first months of life. Birch et al. [31] studied infants who were weaned after about 6 weeks of human milk feeding to formula without or with LCPs and found poorer visual acuity at 17, 26 and 52 weeks of age in the infants who received no LCPs. Similarly, Hoffman et al. [32] observed faster maturation of evoked visual potentials at 1 year of age in infants supplemented from 4 months of age. Moreover, recently, it was demonstrated that early LCP supplementation may influence both the presence of specific immune cell types and function [33].

As estimation of PUFA and LCP requirements is not easy for healthy infants and children, it is even more difficult to give recommendations for children with cholestasis. Still, one should be aware of the risk of PUFA deficiency, and some case reports appeared describing classical dermatological symptoms of essential fatty acid deficiency [34]. There are several factors that contribute to PUFA and LCP deficiency including low PUFA intake, malabsorption and disturbed metabolism of PUFAs to long-chain derivatives. We reported LCP and PUFA deficiency as expressed by plasma phospholipid levels in spite of adequate PUFA content in the diet of cholestatic infants [35]. Extra PUFA intake may improve fatty acid status (e.g., soybean or rapeseed oil) and, in infancy, it seems it should significantly exceed 10% of total energy.

Supplementation of essential fatty acids may not be sufficient. We were able to show increasing impairment of hepatic PUFA conversion to LCPs with an advancing severity of liver disease; thus, severe cholestasis is a significant risk factor for LCP deficiency even with essential fatty acid supply [36]. LCP supplementation can be required based on dietary products like egg yolk (rich in AA) or fish oil (rich in DHA). Infants may be given conventional LCP-supplemented formulae available for healthy term and preterm infants or dietary supplements. Not only low intake, impaired metabolism and decreased absorption may play a role in PUFA deficiency. Unsaturated fatty acids may undergo lipid peroxidation, and increased lipid peroxidation is observed in cholestasis due to impaired antioxidant defense. Even if we observed high lipid peroxide levels and low vitamin E concentrations we were not able to show any direct relationship between PUFAs and lipid peroxides [37, 38]. Profound LCP deficiency may develop in advanced cholestatic liver disease and it can be difficult to correct. It was documented that even 1 year after liver transplantation, the LCP status is not entirely reversed [39]. At the moment, there are no studies showing functional effects of LCP supplementation in children with cholestasis and we cannot give strong recommendations on PUFA and LCP supplementation. It is reasonable in clinical practice to use PUFA-rich vegetable oils and/or egg yolk as dietary supplements to increase energy density and PUFA intake. In infants with cholestasis who receive regular infant formulae and do not require MCT-enriched feeds, LCP-supplemented infant formulae may be used [3].

Vitamins

Lipid-soluble vitamin malabsorption seems to be the major nutritional problem and very specific to cholestasis. Some other factors may also contribute to low lipid-soluble vitamin levels like utilization of vitamin E due to increased free radical formation. Some lipid-soluble vitamins can be efficiently supplemented (vitamins A, D and K), while vitamin E supplementation may cause significant problems. In severe cholestatic liver disease, the oral route of vitamin supplementation may not be sufficient, and parenteral formulations should be considered.

Vitamin A Deficiency

Vitamin A deficiency presents with dry skin, xerophthalmia and night blindness. Serum levels are often used to estimate vitamin A status but they do not correctly reflect vitamin A status. A useful indicator of vitamin A status is the plasma retinol/retinol-binding protein molar ratio [calculated as serum retinol (ng/dl)/serum retinol-binding protein (mg/dl) × 0.0734]. Ratios exceeding 0.8 point to normal vitamin A status. Vitamin A liver metabolism is usually preserved in cholestatic patients [40, 41]. Higher ratios can be associated with toxicity including liver fibrosis, hypercalcemia, pseudotumor cerebri and painful bone lesions. Vitamin A toxicity can be well documented from plasma levels of vitamin A esters. As vitamin A can be toxic, one may consider β-carotene supplementation as a precursor of vitamin A. It is also a lipid-soluble substance that is involved in the protection of membranes against free radical injury complementary to vitamin E and it can be safely used as a supplement in patients with liver disease, contrary to vitamin A supplementation. There is good evidence from in vitro studies that β-carotene is a potent antioxidant that may alleviate the toxic effect of bile acids on liver cells [42]. Also, β-carotene deficiency was reported in adults with prolonged cholestasis [43]. We recently reported low β-carotene levels in children with cholestasis that may be related to poor absorption of this substance from the gut (data ready for publication).

Vitamin D Deficiency

Vitamin D deficiency may also easily develop in prolonged cholestasis. Breastfed infants are at a higher risk, as breast milk contains low amounts of vitamin D. Symptoms of profound vitamin D deficiency can be rarely observed – like hypocalcemia, hypophosphatemia, muscle hypotonia and rickets. In severe liver disease, it is not only poor vitamin D absorption which is responsible for poor availability of vitamin D but also impaired metabolism in the liver can play a significant role. This is why vitamin D is not used to correct a deficiency but instead its metabolite 25-hydroxycholecalciferol (25-OH-D). One should be aware that vitamin D supplementation alone is not effective, and calcium and phosphorus should be given simultaneously. However, treatment with vitamin D does not always prove successful in improving the bone disturbance [44]. Sunlight exposure can be of some help but it is not sufficient. The best indicator of vitamin D status in cholestasis is 25-OH-D serum concentration; levels of 20 ng/ml and less are regarded as extremely low, and the optimal values in healthy subjects are discussed. Concentrations significantly exceeding 25 ng/ml can be regarded desirable. The simple indicator of hypocalcemia can also be used – the urinary calcium/creatinine ratio should be <0.25. However, there is no direct correlation between severity of osteopenia and serum levels of 25(OH)-vitamin D and 1,25(OH)2-vitamin D in either infants or older children with cholestasis. Decreased bone mineralization in childhood cholestasis is a disease process that begins early in infancy, rapidly worsens with increasing age and hepatic dysfunction, and remains relatively stable in children with more stable liver disease [44]. Vitamin D toxicity is seldom reported and includes hypercalcemia and pseudotumor cerebri. Liver transplantation seems to correct osteopenia and vitamin D deficiency. In infants and children younger than 2 years with chronic cholestasis, the bone mineral content normalizes approximately 11 months after orthotopic liver transplantation. This normalization was preceded by a sustained period of normal serum 25-OH-D levels [45].

Vitamin E Deficiency

Vitamin E deficiency seems to be a major problem in prolonged cholestasis which is difficult to correct in some cholestatic diseases. Marked vitamin E deficiency in children with chronic cholestasis leads to neurological degeneration. The most important role of vitamin E is its antioxidative function as an oxygen-free radical scavenger. Insufficient availability of this vitamin may predispose to peroxidation, including that of unsaturated fatty acids, which disrupts the function of central and peripheral nervous system cell membranes. The consequences of vitamin E avitaminosis are particularly serious in children. The initially subtle neurological changes may, after some years, lead to irreversible damage. The neurological signs related to vitamin E deficiency usually include peripheral neuropathy, ophthalmoplegia, ataxia, impaired vibratory sensation and degenerative lesions of the retina. The first signs in the form of disappearance of deep tendon reflexes can manifest themselves relatively early. The nervous system lesions are similar to those observed in other diseases with vitamin E deficiency, such as abetalipoproteinemia, Anderson's disease and familial, selective isolated vitamin E deficiency [46–48].

In many children with cholestasis, it is not possible to obtain improvement in vitamin E status with oral, fat-soluble preparations, which makes it necessary to resort to painful intramuscular injections. Sokol et al. [49–51] reported on the beneficial effect of a new, water-soluble oral vitamin E preparation that corrects α-tocopheryl serum levels and improves existing neurological defects in children with cholestasis. TPGS (d-α-tocopheryl polyethylene glycol 1000 succinate, Eastman Chemical Products Inc., Kingsport, Tenn., USA, or Orphan Europe, Paris, France) is a water-soluble succinic acid ester of vitamin E bound to polyethylene glycol 1000, which can form micelles without the involvement of bile acids. We also reported on the effects of TPGS therapy which quickly normalized serum vitamin E levels but did not improve the increased lipid peroxidation and poor PUFA status [37]. Coadministration of other fat-soluble vitamins in patients with cholestasis can be concerned [52]. Vitamin E therapy monitoring relies on the vitamin E/total lipid ratio (normal >0.8 mg/g but with plasma vitamin E <30 μg/ml). Toxicity is unusual.

Vitamin K Deficiency

Vitamin K deficiency may be an early sign of fat malabsorption in cholestasis [1] resulting in hemorrhagic disease. Important conclusions came from Dutch and Danish national biliary atresia registries. A daily dose of 25 μg of vitamin K failed to prevent bleedings in apparently healthy infants with unrecognized cholestasis because of biliary atresia. One milligram of weekly oral prophylaxis offered significantly higher protection to these infants and was of similar efficacy as 2 mg of intramuscular prophylaxis at birth [53]. In clinical practice, high-dose oral vitamin K every week or every 3 days is used for prevention of bleeding. For treatment of a significant prothrombin time, increased intravenous vitamin K management is the best option. Konakion MM (Roche) seems to be a formulation (vitamin K compound solubilized in glycocholate and lecithin) which efficiently and safely corrects vitamin K deficiency [54].

Vitamin K deficiency can be detected by high international normalized ratio values (increased prothrombin time) which is corrected by parenteral vitamin K administration. PIVKA II (protein induced in the absence of vitamin K), measured by ELISA assay, seems to be a better indicator than prothrombin time (PIVKA II >3 ng/ml reflects vitamin K deficiency) but it is not commonly available.

Water-soluble vitamins should also be supplemented as malabsorption of nutrients may also cause water-soluble vitamin deficiency. Moreover, antioxidants may decrease as they are utilized in protection against high peroxide formation. Single nutrient deficiency, like vitamin C, can be even more profound if combined with low levels of other antioxidants (e.g., vitamin E). In chronic cholestasis, it is advised to use twice the recommended dietary allowance for water-soluble vitamins [3], but in some circumstances, much higher doses of particular vitamins are needed [4]. Low levels of minerals and trace elements were documented in children with cholestasis. Supplements of selenium, zinc, calcium and magnesium

Table 2. Lipid-soluble vitamins in the management of cholestatic children

Lipid-soluble vitamin	Daily requirement	Method of administration
Vitamin A	<10 kg: 5,000 IU >10 kg: 10,000 IU IM: 50,000 IU	oral
Vitamin D	25-OH-D: 2–5 μg/kg IM: 30,000 IU, 1–3 monthly	oral/IM
Vitamin E	TPGS 25 IU/kg IM: 10 mg/kg (max. 200 mg) every 3 weeks	oral
Vitamin K	2 mg/day weekly 5–10 kg: 5 mg >10 kg: 10 mg IM: 5–10 mg every 2 weeks	oral IM

According to Baker et al. [3]. IM = Intramuscular; max. = maximum.

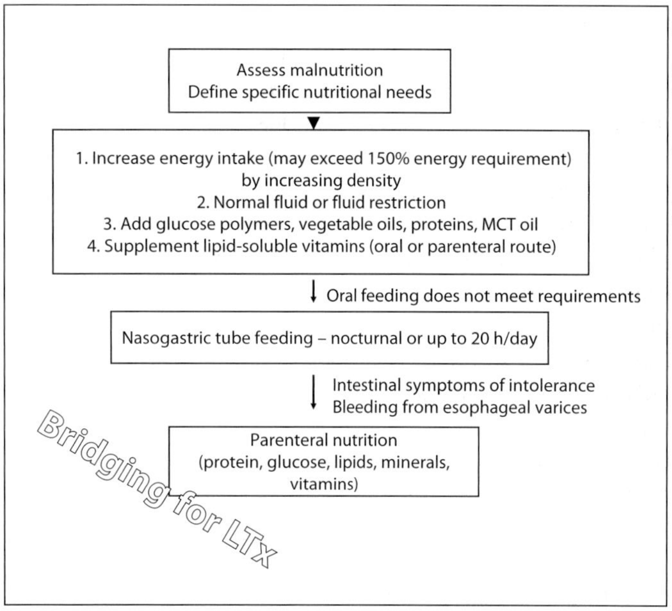

Color version available online

Fig. 2. Feeding algorithm for children with cholestatic liver disease.

should be given as guided by plasma levels [3]. Selenium and zinc are important antioxidants. Iron may enhance oxidative stress and fibrogenesis in patients with liver disease [55]. Thus, iron should not be supplemented on a regular basis. Iron deficiency does not seem to be a common problem in cholestasis. Liver transplantation seems to correct most of the deficiencies and antioxidant status and restores such capacities except for glutathione (table 2) [56].

Oral, Enteral and Parenteral Route of Administration

The oral route is preferable only if sufficient energy and nutrient supply can be secured. Commercial preparations should be used for oral feeding and a well-balanced diet should be obtained under control of a dietician. The feeds should be palatable. Energy-dense preparations can be used to increase energy intake.

In advanced liver disease, especially if a fast catch-up growth is required before liver transplantation, nasogastric tube feeding can be the best option. Bolus feeding cannot always be tolerated. Continuous infusion rate obtained by a pump for up to 20 h a day can solve many problems occurring with tube feeding, like vomiting. Night-time nasogastric tube feeding is another option: the child is allowed to eat ad libitum during the day and receives extra energy when sleeping. The daily preparation of the solutions requires involvement of dieticians. The risk of bacterial contamination of feeds should be a concern. Percutaneous endoscopic gastrostomy is not a common way of nutrient supply because of risk of variceal bleeding.

Parenteral nutrition is needed in a very small percentage of patients as usually the absorptive function of the gastrointestinal tract is preserved. Vomiting, bloating, diarrhea and other complications may cause severe problems in oral and enteral feeding. If energy intake is too low for the requirements, partial parenteral nutrition may improve the nutritional status. Still, the safety of this method of nutritional therapy is strongly related to the experience of the clinical center. The standards of parenteral nutrition in cholestasis are similar as for other indications.

Standard amino acid solutions are used, and no benefit of branched-chain amino acids was documented [57]. Also, lipids are well tolerated. We assessed safety of LCT and MCT/LCT lipid infusions in short-term parenteral nutrition in cholestatic children and we found a good metabolic tolerance of both intravenously infused emulsions in infants with cholestasis. As DHA seems to play a major role in brain development, LCT emulsions may be the optimal source of PUFAs (they contain more PUFAs than MCT/LCT emulsions) for infants with chronic cholestasis if given short term. Our results do not show any risk of increased lipid peroxidation with lipid infusions. Plasma lipid concentrations were not changed by either of the lipid emulsions used [58].

Guimber et al. [59] also reported on safety of parenteral nutrition given to cholestatic children. He observed an increase in Z scores for weight for age and weight for height with no significant change in parameters of liver synthetic function in 7 children with liver disease. The significant increase in bilirubin was probably related to the natural course of the liver disease or could be partially explained by parenteral nutrition. Even if prolonged parenteral nutrition is a risk factor of cholestasis in patients who do not present primary liver disease, this method of nutritional therapy can be used as a 'bridging' for liver transplantation.

Conclusions

Cholestatic liver disease deserves special attention concerning nutrition and nutritional support. Nutritional status should be assessed, and specific nutritional needs should be defined before nutritional therapy can be started. The basic principle of the nutritional management is to correct the nutritional status with additional supply of energy proteins, carbohydrates, lipids and lipid-soluble vitamins. As liver disease progresses to liver failure in many chronic cholestatic diseases, nutritional therapy can be often regarded as 'bridging' for liver transplantation to improve prognosis. Thus, invasive nutritional support is justified in severe liver disease which usually includes nocturnal nasogastric tube feeding or even parenteral nutrition (fig. 2).

References

1 Ijland MM, Pereira RR, Cornelissen EAM: Incidence of late vitamin K deficiency bleeding in newborns in the Netherlands in 2005: evaluation of the current guideline. Eur J Pediatr 2008;167:165–169.

2 Chin SE, Shepherd RW, Thomas BJ, et al: The nature of malnutrition in children with end-stage liver disease awaiting orthotopic liver transplantation. Am J Clin Nutr 1992;56: 164–168.

3 Baker A, Stevenson R, Dhawan A, et al: Guidelines for nutritional care for infants with cholestatic liver disease before liver transplantation. Pediatr Transplant 2007;11: 825–834.

4 Samonte V, Sherman P, Taylor G, et al: Scurvy diagnosed in a paediatric liver transplant patient awaiting combined kidney and liver transplantation. Pediatr Transplant 2008;12: 363–367.

5 Socha P, Litwin M: Editorial to: Scurvy diagnosed in a pediatric liver transplant awaiting combined kidney and liver transplantation. Pediatr Transplant 2008;12:257–260.

6 Heymsfield SB, Waki M, Reinus J: Are patients with chronic liver disease hypermetabolic? Hepatology 1990;11:502–505.

7 Greer R, Lehnert M, Lewindon P, et al: Body composition and components of energy expenditure in children with end-stage liver disease. J Pediatr Gastroenterol Nutr 2003; 36:358–363.

8 Holt RI, Miell JP, Jones JS, et al: Nasogastric feeding enhances nutritional status in paediatric liver disease but does not alter circulating levels of IGF-I and IGF-binding proteins. Clin Endocrinol 2000;52:217–224.

9 Walkowiak J, Jankowska I, Pawlowska J, et al: Exocrine pancreatic function in children with progressive familial intrahepatic cholestasis type 2. J Pediatr Gastroenterol Nutr 2006;42:416–418.

10 Nagasaka H, Yorifuji T, Egawa H, et al: Evaluation of risk for atherosclerosis in Alagille syndrome and progressive familial intrahepatic cholestasis: two congenital cholestatic diseases with different lipoprotein metabolisms. J Pediatr 2005;146:329–335.

11 Sokol RJ, Stall C: Anthropometric evaluation of children with chronic liver disease. Am J Clin Nutr 1990;52:203–208.

12 Trocki O, Wotton MJ, Cleghorn GJ, Shepherd RW: Value of total body potassium in assessing the nutritional status of children with end-stage liver disease. Ann NY Acad Sci 2000;904:400–405.

13 Chongsrisawat V, Ruttanamongkol P, Chaiwatanarat T, et al: Bone density and 25-hydroxyvitamin D level in extrahepatic biliary atresia. Pediatr Surg Int 2001;17:604–608.

14 Graham GG, MacLean WC, Brown KH, et al: Protein requirements of infants and children: growth during recovery from malnutrition. Pediatrics 1996;97:499–505.

15 Tomkins A, Garlick PJ, Schofield WN, Waterlow JC: The combined effect of infection and malnutrition on protein metabolism in children. Clin Sci 1983;65:313–324.

16 Sokal EM, Baudoux MC, Collette E, et al: Branched chain amino acids improve body composition and nitrogen balance in a rat model of extra-hepatic biliary atresia. Pediatr Res 1996;40:66–71.

17 Chin SE, Shepherd RW, Thomas BJ, et al: The nature of malnutrition in children with end-stage liver disease awaiting orthotopic liver transplantation. Am J Clin Nutr 1992;56: 164–168.

18 Koletzko B, Demmelmair H, Socha P: Nutritional support of infants and children: supply and metabolism of lipids. Baillieres Clin Gastroenterol 1998;12:671–696.

19 Beath S, Hooley, Willis K, et al: Long chain triacylglycerol malabsorption and pancreatic function in children with protein energy malnutrition complicating severe liver disease. Proc Nutr Soc 1993;52:252A.

20 Bach AC, Babayan V: Medium-chain triglycerides: an update. Am J Clin Nutr 1982;36: 950–962.

21 Kaufman SS, Murray ND, Wood RP, et al: Nutritional support for the infants with extrahepatic biliary atresia. J Pediatr 1987;10: 679–685.

22 Rebouche CJ, Panagides DD, Nelson SE: Role of carnitine in utilization of dietary medium-chain triglycerides by term infants. Am J Clin Nutr 1990;52:820–824.

23 Kaufmann SS, Scrivner DJ, Murray ND, et al: Influence of portagen and pregestimil on essential fatty acid status in infantile liver disease. Pediatrics 1992;89:151–154.

24 Bach A, Schirardin H, Bauer M, Weryha A: Ketogenic response to medium-chain triglyceride load in the rat. J Nutr 1977;107: 1863–1870.

25 Beath SV, Johnson S, Willis KD, et al: Growth and luminal fat solubilisation in cholestatic infants on medium chain triglyceride (MCT). J Pediatr Gastroenterol Nutr 1996;22:443.

26 Koletzko B, Agostoni C, Carlson SE, et al: Long chain polyunsaturated fatty acids (LC-PUFA) and perinatal development. Acta Paediatr 2001;90:460–464.
27 Koletzko B: Fats for brains. Eur J Clin Nutr 1992;46:S51–S62.
28 Demmelmair H, von Schenck U, Behrendt E, et al: Estimation of arachidonic acid synthesis in full term neonates using natural variation of C13 content. J Pediatr Gastroenterol Nutr 1995;21:31–36.
29 Simmer K: Longchain polyunsaturated fatty acid supplementation in infants born at term (Cochrane Review); in The Cochrane Library, Issue 3. Cichester, Wiley, 2004.
30 Uauy R, Hoffman DR, Mena P, et al: Term infant studies of DHA and ARA supplementation on neurodevelopment: results of randomized controlled trials. J Pediatr 2003; 143:S17–S25.
31 Birch EE, Hoffman DR, Castañeda YS, et al: A randomized controlled trial of long-chain polyunsaturated fatty acid supplementation of formula in term infants after weaning at 6 wk of age. Am J Clin Nutr 2002;75:570–580.
32 Hoffman DR, Birch EE, Castañeda YS, et al: Visual function in breast-fed term infants weaned to formula with or without long-chain polyunsaturates at 4 to 6 months: a randomized clinical trial. J Pediatr 2003;142: 669–677.
33 Field CJ, Van Aerde JE, Robinson LE, Clandinin MT: Effect of providing a formula supplemented with long-chain polyunsaturated fatty acids on immunity in full-term neonates. Br J Nutr 2008;99:91–99.
34 Levy J, DeFelice A, Lepage G: Essential fatty acid deficiency mimicking porphyria cutanea tarda in a patient with chronic cholestasis. J Pediatr Gastroenterol Nutr 1990;10: 242–245.
35 Socha P, Koletzko B, Świątkowska E, et al: Essential fatty acid metabolism in infants with cholestasis. Acta Pediatr 1998;87:278–283.
36 Socha P, Koletzko B, Pawlowska P, Socha J: Essential fatty acid status in children with cholestasis, in relation to serum bilirubin concentration. J Pediatr 1997;131:700–706.
37 Socha P, Koletzko B, Pawlowska J, et al: Treatment of cholestatic children with water-soluble vitamin E (alpha-tocopheryl polyethylene glycol succinate): effects on serum vitamin E, lipid peroxides, and polyunsaturated fatty acids. J Pediatr Gastroenterol Nutr 1997;24:189–193.
38 Socha P, Koletzko B, Świątkowska E, et al: Essential fatty acid metabolism in infants with cholestasis. Acta Pediatr 1998;87:278–283.
39 Lapillonne A, Hakme C, Mamoux V, et al: Effects of liver transplantation on long-chain polyunsaturated fatty acid status in infants with biliary atresia. J Pediatr Gastroenterol Nutr 2000;30:528–532.
40 Hochman J, Balistreri WF: Neonatal cholestasis: differential diagnosis, evaluation and management; in Balistreri WF, Ohi R, Todani T, Tsuchida Y (eds): Hepatobiliary, Pancreatic and Splenic Disease in Children. Amsterdam, Elsevier, 1997.
41 Amedée-Manesme O, Furr HC, Alvarez F, et al: Biochemical indicators of vitamin A depletion in children with cholestasis. Hepatology 1985;5:1143–1148.
42 Gumpricht E, Dahl R, Devereaux MW, Sokol RJ: β-Carotene prevents bile acid-induced cytotoxicity in rat hepatocyte: evidence for an antioxidant and anti-apoptotic role of β-carotene in vitro. Pediatr Res 2004;55:814–821.
43 Leon AM, Ahmed S, Aleynik SI, et al: Carotenoids and tocopherols in various hepatobiliary conditions. J Hepatol 1995;23:550–556.
44 Argao EA, Specker BL, Heubi JE: Bone mineral content in infants and children with chronic cholestatic liver disease. Pediatrics 1993;91:1151–1154.
45 Argao EA, Balistreri WF, Hollis BW, et al: Effect of orthotopic liver transplantation on bone mineral content and serum vitamin D metabolites in infants and children with chronic cholestasis. Hepatology 1994;20: 598–603.
46 Anderson CM, Townley RR, Freeman JP: Unusual causes of steatorrhea in infancy and childhood. Med J Aust 1961;11:617–621.
47 Nasr SZ, O'Leary MH, Hillermeier C: Correction of vitamin E deficiency with fat-soluble versus water-miscible preparations of vitamin E in patients with cystic fibrosis. J Pediatr 1993;122:810–812.
48 Sokol RJ, Kayden HJ, Bettis DB, et al: Isolated vitamin E deficiency in the absence of fat malabsorption – familial and sporadic cases: characterization and investigations of causes. J Lab Clin Med 1988;11:548–559.
49 Sokol RJ, Butler-Simon N, Conner C, et al: Multicenter trial of d-M-tocopheryl polyethylene glycol 1000 succinate for treatment of vitamin E deficiency in children with chronic cholestasis. Gastroenterology 1993;104: 1727–1735.
50 Sokol RJ, Heubi JE, Butler-Simon N, et al: Treatment of vitamin E deficiency during chronic childhood cholestasis with oral d-T-tocopheryl polyethylene glycol-1000-succinate. Gastroenterology 1987;93:975–985.
51 Sokol RJ, Guggenheim MA, Iannaccone ST, et al: Improved neurologic function following long-term correction of vitamin E deficiency in children with chronic cholestasis. N Engl J Med 1985;313:1580–1586.
52 Argao EA, Heubi JE: Fat-soluble vitamin deficiency in infants and children. Curr Opin Pediatr 1993;5:562–566.
53 van Hasselt PM, de Koning TJ, Kvist N, et al: The Netherlands Study Group for Biliary Atresia Registry. Prevention of vitamin K deficiency bleeding in breastfed infants: lessons from the Dutch and Danish biliary atresia registries. Pediatrics 2008;121:e857–e863.
54 Amedée-Manesme O, Lambert WE, Alagille D, De Leenheer AP: Pharmacokinetics and safety of a new solution of vitamin K_1 in children with cholestasis. J Pediatr Gastroenterol Nutr 1992;14:160–165.
55 Bonkovsky HL, Banner BF, Lambrecht RW, Rubin RB: Iron in liver diseases other than haemochromatosis. Semin Liver Dis 1996; 16:65–82.
56 Wierzbicka A, Pawłowska J, Socha P, et al: Lipid, carbohydrate metabolism, and antioxidant status in children after liver transplantation. Transplant Proc 2007;39:1523–1525.
57 Plauth M, Merli M, Weimann A, et al: ESPEN guidelines for nutrition in liver disease and transplantation. Clin Nutr 1997;16:43–45.
58 Socha P, Koletzko B, Demmelmair H, et al: Short-term effects of parenteral nutrition of cholestatic infants with lipid emulsions based on medium-chain and long-chain triacylglycerols. Nutrition 2007;23:121–126.
59 Guimber D, Michaud L, Ategbo S, et al: Experience of parenteral nutrition for nutritional rescue in children with severe liver disease following failure of enteral nutrition. Pediatr Transplant 1999;3:139–145.